**DO NOT REMOVE
CARDS FROM POCKET**

An Older Woman's
HEALTH GUIDE

The Older Woman's Health Project was conducted under grants made to the Division of Gerontology, New York University Medical Center.

An Older Woman's HEALTH GUIDE

Joan Mintz, Director
The Older Woman's
Health Project

written by
Mary Egginton
Maryann Kunigonis
Joan Mintz
Dorothy Roser

G.K. HALL &CO.
Boston, Massachusetts
1986

Published in Large Print by arrangement
with McGraw-Hill Book Company.

British Commonwealth rights courtesy of
June Hall Literary Agency.

G. K. Hall Large Print Book Series.

Set in 16 pt Plantin.

Library of Congress Cataloging in Publication Data
Main entry under title:

   An Older woman's health guide.

   (G.K. Hall large print book series)
   1. Aged women—Care and hygiene. 2. Aged
women—Care and hygiene—United States.
3. Aged women—United States—Social conditions.
4. Aged women—Services for—United States—
Directories. 5. Large type books. I. Mintz,
Joan. II. Egginton, Mary.
[RA778.034   1986]   613'.04244   85-24769
ISBN 0-8161-3985-7 (lg. print)

To the older women whose friendship, wisdom,
and enthusiasm made possible the writing of this book.

CONTENTS

A *n Older Woman's Health Guide* is an answer to
a need that has become increasingly apparent
to professionals concerned with aging as well as to
older women themselves. Older women represent
the majority of people over 65 in the United States,
yet their specific physical and mental health problems have rarely been differentiated from those of
their male counterparts, and have largely been neglected.

The Older Woman's Health Project, initiated in
1979 with support from private foundations and
corporations, first ran a series of health education
classes with a dual purpose: (1) to assist older wom-
en toward better health through education and (2)
to learn from participants about health problems of
particular concern to older women. Because the
classes were limited to New York City residents, the
project, with the assistance of our Advisory Committee, also devised a questionnaire and distributed
it nationally through approximately two hundred
organizations and interested individuals.

From the responses of the class participants, the
answers to over one thousand questionnaires, the
input from our Advisory Committee, consultations
with other organizations, and an exhaustive search

of the literature, this *Guide* was planned and implemented.

Our thanks go to the Chatlos Foundation for an initial grant to start the Older Woman's Health Project followed by two years' funding to sustain it; to the New York Foundation for funding the research and writing of the *Guide;* to Chesebrough-Pond, Inc., Conoco, and Pfizer Pharmaceutical for supplementary contributions; to the members of our Advisory Committee, our colleagues in the field, and our devoted staff for their advice and support; and last to New York University Medical Center, of which this program is a part.

Mary Egginton
Maryann Kunigonis
Joan Mintz
Dorothy Roser

This is a book that deals not with sickness, but with health. Although the authors have written about a variety of different physical problems that may afflict elderly women, they approach the subject with something that feels like a smile. All of the many questions that trouble those of us who are classified as "elderly" by our society are dealt with. We are reminded how much well-being can be augmented by sound social relationships, by lack of stress, and by a life style that is both physically and mentally active.

There has long been a recognition of the fact that the elderly population is made up in large part of women. Women outlive men by at least eight years. Those extra years are too often wasted, arid, and meaningless. Women too often believe the stereotypes that society has assigned to them. They see themselves as physically unattractive, as having lost all appeal for men, as being a burden to their families, and as suffering from such embarrassing problems as loss of hearing, weakened eyesight, and mental confusion. Stereotypes are false, but the conviction of masses of women that they are true means that they have become self-fulfilling prophecies. That's why this book carries such an important message. It explodes the myth and it gives constructive answers to those aspects of the stereotypes that may affect individuals.

Perhaps the next generations of the elderly will have experienced a world that will make old age easier. The present generation is pioneering. It is the first generation that in large numbers has lived past the age of eighty. Twenty years ago golden wedding anniversaries were reported in the papers as "phenomena." Today they are far from uncommon. Twenty years ago an active, intelligent involved woman in her nineties was newsworthy. Today centenarians who are still functioning rationally no longer astonish us.

Because so few of the present generation of older women were in the labor force, Social Security payments for this generation are low. The next generation of women who reach the upper age levels will, in a growing number of cases, have had college educations and careers. The effect of this change will be interesting to watch.

In the meantime it is distressing that so little has been written about *life* in the age period of sixty-five to eighty-five and above. So much, on the other hand, has been written about illness and death, on how to handle the frail elderly, and on how to deal with fading mental ability. There is no reason to suppose that the last twenty years of life are any less important or meaningful to human beings than the first twenty. There have been, of course, a great many books written about those first twenty years of life. Studies of emotional and physical growth of infants, studies of the learning capacities of young children, research into adolescence—projects that deal with development in all childhood phases are common. There are bookshelves in the libraries full of volumes dealing in detail with all of the first years of life. Certainly no one can quarrel with the importance of those years. The way in which our society handles its children and its young adults has a permanent impact on the shape of that society. On the other hand all life and living is important, and there is no reason why the twenty years from sixty-five to eighty-five should be any less meaningful, nor is there any reason why life for older people should be less precious and less rich. It is time for us to appreciate that every period of life has meaning, and everyone is entitled to live in each of these periods to the fullest. There is a wealth of experience and knowledge to be gained from insuring that our older women are enabled to play an active role.

It is this message that is carried, subtly, in *An Older Woman's Health Guide*. The book itself covers far more than questions of health goals, or health problems. It is a complete travel guide for the older woman in her journey through the vital years after fifty-five. It includes careful analysis of social and family relationships, of various educational and employment opportunities, of legal resources, money management, and, of course, of health care. It shows women how to be as well as they can be, and better than they dreamed was possible, through exercise, diet, and sound living practices. It gives guidance to women on how to live with loneliness without being lonely, and how to live with grief without allowing it to become devouring.

There is an enormous amount of very practical information contained in this book. It has a great many answers to the questions we want to ask our doctor but that we are reluctant to verbalize because we feel that we are imposing on someone else's valuable time. It is specific about certain types of diseases that are characteristic of aging as well as about the preventions and cures. It is specific too, about opportunities for varied activities that are available to the elderly. Most of all it carries a message of quiet confidence. We, the older women of today, are blazing a trail for the next generations of women who will be following us. For the first time in the history of mankind, or, perhaps, more appropriately, in the case of womenkind, a sizable number of us are experiencing old age. How we view ourselves, how we deal with it personally as well as in relation to our families and our friends, how we cope with shrunken incomes, decreasing circles of friends, loss of loved ones, housing problems, loneliness and the need to deal with complicated financial and legal problems for which we were never prepared—all these are the subjects of this book. They are also subjects that are becoming important to the entire society. Not only the elderly but those who have questions about elderly parents or those who are wise enough to wonder about their own futures will find answers in *An Older Woman's Health Guide*. The authors have made a major contribution to our understanding of old age and to our potential for living wisely and well.

Elinor Guggenheimer
Chairman of the Council of Senior Centers and
  Services
Member of Technical Committee for White
  House Conference on Aging, 1981

ONE

What
Is Health?

Health, to many of us, is an abstract idea which is taken for granted until it is lost. We speak often of being and remaining healthy and say things like "Smoking is bad for your health" or "Vegetables and fruits are part of a healthy diet." But what exactly is "health"? Are you healthy if you are not sick? Is health dependent on social and environmental factors as well as on physical and emotional ones? Are there different levels of health? Can one be healthy while having a chronic disease?

Health is more than lack of illness. It is a positive state involving physical well-being, emotional satisfaction, and having feelings of self-worth and contentment and a sense of control over the conditions and experiences of life. It is affected by social and family relationships, culture, and environment. It is not a static state but changes in response to shifts in all these factors. One can feel very healthy at times and less healthy, although not ill, at others.

In this book we will look at "health" in its wholeness—physical, mental, and social, as it applies to older women—and outline some specific ways to maintain it. In order to do this, we must determine who we older women are, where we live, what we do, and how we feel about ourselves. In subsequent chapters we suggest ways to stay physically and mentally healthy, to deal with disease and the health care system, and to maintain our changing relationship with others in the most rewarding ways. The final chapter describes some alternatives to traditional health care. All the resources we have been able to discover to help older women stay well and happy are listed in the Appendices.

WHO ARE WE OLDER WOMEN?

At any age we are the sum of what we have been— a complicated mix of our genes and our social environment, our life experience and our individual reactions to it. For we older women in the 1980s for whom this book is written, it is indeed a mix. We have lived through wars, depressions, inflations, recessions, and in our "spare time" have been wives, mothers, grandparents, friends, students, employers, and almost always homemakers. Probably in the entire recorded history of mankind there have not been so many vast changes in peoples' conditions as have taken place in our lifetimes. For instance:

Women 55 to 65 today were born between 1925 and 1915. They missed World War I and were children or adolescents during the Great Depression of the 1930s. The older ones' marriages may well have been profoundly affected by World War II, and their middle years passed during the subsequent history-making events: the atomic, space, and electronic ages; the civil rights and feminist movements; the political assassinations; the Vietnam War; confrontation and the problems of the drug culture and the unknowns of the 1980s.

Women 65 to 75 were born between 1915 and 1905. Some will remember their childhood during World War I. Their fathers or family friends may have been casualties of that bloody "war to end wars." With the Great Depression the most significant public event in their lives, they may have been deeply scarred as adolescents by poverty or fear of poverty. The older members of this age group may have watched their husbands or "intendeds" hopelessly seeking employment. Then they were in the midst of the turmoil of World War II; some were widowed and some childless because of their husbands' absences during peak childbearing years. Homemaking was a mad scramble for food rations, transportation—just survival. Those who could went to work. These were the days of "Rosie, the Riveter," possibly the pioneer feminist of the twentieth century. These women may have been positively affected by the economic "good times" that followed the end of that era, and most of them were aware of the growing social unrest of the 1950s, 1960s, and 1970s.

Women 75 to 85 were born between 1895 and 1905, children of the Victorian era. Queen Victoria of England died in 1901, and her mores, along with our "puritan ethic," deeply affected the ways of her time. These women were born when social values and restrictions were stratified and rigid—were expected to last forever—when "the rich got richer and the poor got poorer," and society seemed not to care. Television and radio did not exist, and the wireless and the telephone were in a rudimentary stage.

Elinor Guggenheimer, now Chairman of the Council of Senior Centers and Services of New York City, who has formerly held many key posts in the human services and is herself a "senior citizen," said at a recent conference for the mature woman that "we are fat and thin and bright and stupid and active and talented and dull and boring; we are mean and loving and greedy and generous and healthy and unhealthy. We have been molded by genetics, the society and our varied life experiences." In short, we are simply individuals who have been around for a while, and most of us have profited from our experiences.

Viewed statistically by social scientists, we do have traits and trends in common. For the purposes of this book, we are limiting our observations to women because women's problems are different from those of their male counterparts at any age; to women over 55 because childbearing years and mid-life crises are mostly over, with a special focus on those 65 and over because that is a magic age at which society labels all of us as "older."

We are the fastest-growing sector of the population. In 1900 there were about 3 million people (male and female) over 65, 4 percent of the population. Today there are 25 million people over 65, representing 11 percent of the whole. Women constitute the vast majority of this sector. (Black women constitute 8 percent of this number.) Between 1964 and 1970 alone, the number of women over 65 increased 42 percent as compared with 18 percent for the entire population.

Women live longer than men. Statistically, today, a 65-year-old woman can expect to live 17.5 more years; a man of the same age, 13.4 more years. (A black woman can expect to live some fewer years than a white woman.) In 1977 there were 3 women over 65 for every 2 men, and the ratio increases annually. Ms. Guggenheimer commented wryly that in our age group "men are in such demand that they run the risk of being killed in the rush, thereby further exaggerating the ratio."

One-third of us older women live alone, 53 percent as widows. The likelihood of our remarrying is slight, since there are 5.5 times as many widows as there are widowers, and many of the latter with society's blessing marry younger women, whereas marriages the other way around are seriously frowned upon.

Because women over 65 in the 1980s were largely shortchanged educationally (only 8 percent with four or more years of college) and did not enter the work force in large numbers until after World War II, many are now deprived economically, with low Social Security and private pension benefits.

Tish Sommers, coordinator of the Task Force of Older Women of the National Organization of Women (NOW), in her 1975 testimony before a House Select Committee on Aging lists the Social Security inequities against women.

When the system was introduced we were supposed to be homemakers with our earnings of very secondary importance . . . [but] in 1970, 38% of the workforce were females. The divorce rate has doubled between 1960 and 1973 . . . (with one-fourth of the divorces after more than 15 years of marriage . . . leaving more women alone without financial support). Sex discrimination in employment begets sex discrimination in retirement. . . . Women are punished for motherhood. The long periods women are out of the job market show up later in reduced benefits. Pay twice, collect once. . . . When more than one person works in the family, the employed wife may receive no benefit for her payroll tax contribution and no credit for labor in the home. The widow's gap comes about when the youngest child reaches 18, and the widow's benefits cease until she reaches 60. The displaced homemaker—a new category of disadvantaged persons . . . widowed, divorced, or separated in their middle years . . . too old to find jobs, too young for Social Security benefits.

She sums up her blacklist with these words: "and what do you have? A classic syndrome of institutionalized sexism. Social Security as it now stands is highly discriminatory against women—not in an abstract 'equal under the law sense' but in the far more real test of how it keeps the wolf from the door."

In a youth-oriented culture, society's perception

of us is unlovely; as portrayed in books, magazines, and the media, we are wrinkled, rigid, asexual, and incompetent. Fortunately, our perception of ourselves is quite different, as will be seen at the close of this chapter.

Statistically, women over 65 are less healthy than men (86 percent of us are said to have some chronic disability), although we live longer. This figure is misleading, however, because, also statistically, women consult health care professionals more regularly than men do and, in the process of diagnosis, may unwittingly become a statistic. However, studies have indicated that women cope with adversity, physical and emotional, better than do men. Obviously, they have had more experience.

These stereotypes do not make an encouraging collage, but we must remember that they *are* stereotypes, and even these are changing as women of all ages become more self-aware, self-reliant, better educated, and more involved in the world of work. As there are more and more of us, our political and social clout increases. Politicians in election years are regular lunchtime visitors at senior centers for the simple reason that older people vote in very large numbers. As awareness of our strength grows, "we get older and better," Guggenheimer remarked.

WHERE DO WE LIVE AND WHAT DO WE DO?

As our numbers increase, so do the numbers of social scientists (as well as politicians) who study us. By selecting sample populations and abstracting pieces of information they discover trends and tendencies about age, geographic location, occupations, health states, and ethnic backgrounds.

We have seen that one-third of us live alone and that 56 percent of us are widows by age 65. Some choose to live with relatives or friends; others go it alone; and still others move to retirement communities or residencies seeking the company and comfort of their peers. The majority of us older people, both black and white, live in cities either because we prefer it or because we have no choice. City life often becomes older people. An older woman, riding on a bus, said of New York: "When I feel low, I go out and walk around. There's always something to see, or someone to talk to or feel sorry for. I love it. I wouldn't change it for all the trees in New England."

Transportation, though sometimes slow and irritating, is there, and we don't have to wait for availability of a friend's or a daughter's car for a trip to the supermarket. Health care and other support systems are near at hand. Though not always the best, they are better than having no independently available support at all. And city dwellers make better neighbors than they are given credit for.

Others love the country and regard city dwellers as creatures loosed from a zoo. Older people tend not to remain in the suburbs, but this trend is changing.

Three-fifths of the black older population still reside in the South, with large concentrations in central cities with the worst housing. Black women who predominate in these ghettos all too often suffer from quadruple jeopardy—racism, sexism, ageism, and poverty.

There is a tendency among us to move to warm climates, if we can afford it. This trend is indicated by the rate of growth of the older population of such places as Arizona, Florida, Hawaii, Nevada, and New Mexico. This urge to move may be motivated by a need to get away from ourselves and our dissatisfactions and as such should be suspect, because "wherever we go, there we are!" In addition, there is more to living than keeping warm, and we will find that it is much hotter *there* when it's hot *here* and that we may not be able to return for any length of time. Although we may find friends in a new locality, they will not be the tried and true ones who can share our memories and put up with our foibles. And we will probably be more isolated from our busy children.

On the other hand, it could be time for a change, stimulation, a new challenge; or a physical disability might be helped by a change in climate. The choice is ours, but it should be a deliberate and careful one.

Our primary occupation may still be "housewife" or "homemaker," and for this reason we often have trouble setting up housekeeping with other women. A woman is usually queen in her own kitchen, modern or primitive, and too many queens can spoil the broth. We tend to treasure our own possessions and want them with us in our own place, which creates additional tensions in multiple living arrangements.

Going back to school (either for vocational upgrading or just for fun) has become a happy trend among us older women.

Some of us are still working and sacrificing at least a portion of our Social Security benefits if we are between 65 and 70 and earn over a specific sum which changes annually. Starting in 1983, people 70 and over can earn any amount without losing benefits, but only 5 percent of people over 70 are gainfully employed.

Some women work part-time maintaining an earned income below the Social Security allowance, thus supplementing their incomes. But unless they are already employed work is hard to find. A segment of our group most often seeking work because they must are divorced women under 62 who have been married less than 10 years and thus are not eligible for their husbands' Social Security either. (Some of these women have coalesced into a group called Displaced Homemakers, which is lobbying for legislation for their own benefit.)

For those of us who do not have to work to live, volunteering can be a very satisfying way to remain involved, busy, and useful. Although the feminist movement of the last quarter century tried to downgrade volunteerism (work without monetary compensation) as a kind of concession or cop-out, its adherents overlooked the fact that they, themselves, as advocates of women's rights were mostly volunteers. The majority of people who volunteer some of their time and energy also work for pay. Often we are not aware that we are volunteering as members of a community group, a library board, even as good friends to a neighbor in need. There are hundreds of informal social arrangements that need volunteers in order to function, as well as the more formalized services in institutional settings. If volunteerism stopped for a day, society would cease to function. So an older woman with time on her hands, or even without it, need feel neither ashamed nor put upon by volunteering in a cause or situation that interests her.

Management of volunteer programs is becoming a legitimate profession, and as a result volunteers are being involved in more and more meaningful activities. We should design our voluntary commitment as carefully as we plan a full-time career and then stick to it. Volunteers who are not reliable are not helping themselves or the program they espouse.

To quote Ms. Guggenheimer once more, "in order to keep healthy, one must remain active—physically, mentally, emotionally. . . . There is strong evidence that those who remain employed either in paying or volunteer jobs that are meaningful (even into the 70's and 80's) are liable to be healthier and happier."

HOW WE SEE OURSELVES

Age (like beauty) is in the eye of the beholder. Few of us see ourselves as "old." Oldness is thrust upon us by outsiders. Recent social legislation in the

United States, designed to answer the needs of special groups including older people, has tended to label us as "old" and, therefore, possibly incapable of dealing effectively with our own lives. This is not the way we see ourselves, as indicated by the following statements regarding their self-image made by participants in our health classes for older women and by respondents to our questionnaires:

"We walk alone in a Noah's Ark world."

"There's a sense of urgency, so much yet to do in life."

"Keep moving—it's hard to hit a moving target."

"If you project inner vitality and a positive self-image, others will find you attractive."

"I forget until I look in the mirror and then it's a shock."

"It's vitally important to forget oneself and concentrate beyond that small circle. To quote Helen Keller on maturity: 'This can be the best stage and the most interesting part of our lives, providing we don't look so long at the closed door that we cannot see the one that is opening.'"

"Absence of work structure on retirement, can be joy, can be difficult."

"Less lonely when alone at home—difference between being lonely and being alone."

"Not caring what others think as much as when

younger—allowing a sense of freedom about life, activities, friends, the new experience of taking care of oneself, instead of everyone else (boss, husband, children), deserving to be good to oneself and not delay pleasures and happiness. Enjoy the time that is left."

These women seemed wonderfully aware of the advantages as well as the disadvantages of being older—independence, more freedom, less responsibility; increased wisdom, knowledge, and patience. The majority were also thinking and planning in positive directions, given the facts of aging—look ahead, keep moving, think about others.

The most frequently voiced problems were coping with loneliness, combating ageism directed particularly toward older women, and coping with the health care system.

TWO

Maintaining Wellness

INTERACTION OF MENTAL AND PHYSICAL HEALTH

M*ens sana in corpore sano,* a healthy mind in a healthy body, describes a two-way street. Physical disease can, and does, adversely affect even the strongest psyche. In the opposite direction, unhealthy mental attitudes can cause a variety of adverse and very real physical symptoms.

Our mental and physical health is our responsibility and our birthright. If a woman determines to do everything in her power to better her physical being through sound, self-imposed living habits—exercise, nutrition, sleep, recreation—the chances are that she will maintain wellness throughout her life. If, however, she has or develops a chronic disability, she may have no choice but to live with it and its limitations. Again, if her environment is detrimental to her health but cannot be changed, she may have to accept that, too.

Older women's increasing longevity and our predisposition to chronic illness together indicate that we need more health information and a greater range of health services. However, since the special health needs of older women have often been ig-

19

nored by the health care system and information services are hard to find, we older women must take a more active role in fulfilling our own health needs, first by learning about health, and second by applying that knowledge to ourselves and to our use of the system.

Fortunately, it has become easier to do this. In recent years, Americans have developed a great interest in improving personal health fitness. People want to know more about exercise, nutrition, stress, environmental pollution, and alternatives to traditional medicine. These topics are enthusiastically discussed in the popular media. However, too much information, some of it contradictory, leads to confusion. Some of it may even be dangerous. It is important to have accurate, sensible information in order to attain our best health.

One outgrowth of this interest in health has been the development of the wholistic health movement. "Wholism," as the word implies, considers the whole person in relation to the environment when determining the state of one's health. It stresses maintaining and improving wellness, the relationship between physical and emotional health, illness prevention, self-help and self-care, and taking responsibility for one's health through increased knowledge about one's body and healthful living. The emphasis is on health—how to maintain and improve it—rather than on illness. We older women should use these same concepts to improve our own health.

One additional thing. We must remember that

medical care is only a part of health care. Medicine tends to focus on illness and its treatment rather than on wellness and its promotion. Treatment of illness is obviously important, but we must also know how to stay well. Other health care professions and disciplines such as nutrition, psychology, nursing, physical therapy, acupuncture, and chiropractic offer a variety of means to improve our health. These should be part of our health plan, and will be discussed elsewhere in this book. We have used the term "health care practitioner" throughout the book to indicate all professionals involved in health care.

NORMAL AGING

Aging is a normal process which begins at birth and ends with death. We do not start "aging" at 30, 40, 50, or 60—we've been aging all along! However, no one ages in exactly the same way. Therefore, changes which occur in one person at 40 may not occur in another person until 55. Also, certain changes may occur in some people but not in others.

A variety of factors affect the physical changes which take place as people get older. Genetic traits inherited from parents and grandparents interact with both life style and environment to affect aging. Research has shown that changes once thought to be inevitable may not be. It is often difficult to separate so-called normal changes from illness. For example, atherosclerosis, the buildup of fatty deposits in the arteries, has been found to be strongly related to diet and smoking rather than a malfunction of aging. We have more control over the aging process than we think. While we cannot change our genes, we can regulate, to varying degrees, such factors as diet, exercise, sleep, stress, smoking, air pollution, and working conditions so that we age as healthfully as possible.

Our attitudes toward growing older are also important. Many women think that physical attractiveness belongs only to the young or that there is no long-term benefit in caring for oneself. Fortunately, ideas like this are changing, and older women are learning to feel good about themselves. Knowing that the myths and stereotypes about older women are just that—myths and stereotypes—promotes a more positive self-image. Health, attractiveness, and vitality are possible at any age.

In this book we will concentrate first on the normal changes which most people experience. Later on we will discuss specific illnesses and conditions which are more prevalent in older people, especially in older women.

Skin

The skin generally becomes drier and less elastic as we age. We perspire less. There is a decrease in the amount of head and body hair, and the hair which remains becomes thinner. These changes make older people more sensitive to cold. Since dry skin may be a problem, it is important to lubricate the skin daily with a moisturizing cream or lotion. These need not be expensive to be useful. Some good examples are cocoa butter and rosewater and glycerine. To be most effective, these products should be applied to damp skin. Baths should be short and taken in warm rather than hot water. Since soap can be very drying, use a minimal amount of a mild soap.

Wrinkles, especially on the face, are bothersome. Skin dryness, inelasticity, repeated use of the muscles of expression ("laugh lines"), and the pull of gravity contribute to wrinkle formation, but the major cause is exposure to the sun.

Even small amounts of sun can cause these skin changes. Long exposure over a period of years leads to premature aging of the skin and increases the risk of skin cancer. So it is wise to limit exposure to the sun and to protect skin while in the sun. A number of creams, lotions, and makeup products contain effective sunscreens like PABA (para-aminobenzoic acid) or sulisobenzene. Read labels to check for these ingredients in the products used. There are degrees of protection from sun, ranging from 1 to 15 in these products. The higher the number, the fewer the sun's rays which get to your skin. The high numbers are particularly recommended for fair-skinned, blue-eyed blondes or redheads.

Eyes

The lens of the eye begins losing its elasticity in the teenage years. This continues into the forties, usually resulting in farsightedness (presbyopia)—difficulty in seeing objects close by with distance vision remaining normal. Consequently, many people over 40 need reading glasses or bifocals.

Ears

It is normal for hearing ability to decrease slightly as one ages. However, this loss usually affects only high tones and does not interfere with normal hearing.

Teeth

Tooth loss and denture wear are *not* a normal part of aging! Unfortunately, life-long neglect results in tooth decay and loss, as well as in diseases of the gums. Certain illnesses and medications also affect the teeth.

Recession of the gums, increased dryness of the mouth, and a decreased sense of taste are normal aging changes as, happily, is *decreased* susceptibility to tooth decay.

Bones and Joints

Older people tend to be shorter than they were when they were young for a number of reasons. The spaces between the vertebrae (bones of the spine) decrease as the cartilage between them shrinks with age, making the vertebrae closer together and the spine shorter. Curvature of the spine can develop as one ages. Poor posture makes us appear shorter than we really are.

Our bones gradually become thinner and more brittle as we age. A low-calcium diet and inactivity can cause this change to progress more rapidly. In some older women this loss of bone mass is severe, leading to a serious condition called osteoporosis. (For a thorough discussion of prevention and treatment see Chapter 4.)

Most people have arthritic changes in their joints which can be seen on x-ray by the time they are 40 and are thought to be the result of wear and tear over the years. At present these changes are considered a part of normal aging, and most people have no symptoms from them. (For more information on arthritis see Chapter 4.)

Uterus, Ovaries, Vagina

Most women stop having menstrual periods by their early fifties. This normal change (menopause) signals the end of a woman's childbearing years. Since this change concerns mid-life rather than older women, it will not be discussed here. However, physical changes do take place at this time which affect a woman's health later in life.

The ovaries and the uterus decrease slightly in size. Estrogen production by the ovaries gradually declines. In the postmenopausal years estrogen is still produced in the body but in much smaller amounts than before menopause. One consequence of this change is vaginal dryness which can cause itching or pain, especially pain during intercourse. Using a water-soluble lubricant such as K-Y Jelly before intercourse helps. (Oil-based lubricants such as petroleum jelly should not be used.) An estrogen cream may be applied to the vagina, but because of the controversy about the safety of estrogen therapy this option frightens many women. Estrogen cream *is* absorbed into the bloodstream. However, the dosage of estrogen in the cream is usually lower than the dosage of estrogen pills, and use is intermittent. The advantages and disadvantages of this treatment, along with the need for such follow-up testing as pap smears, should be thoroughly discussed with your health care practitioner. The cream is available only by prescription. (For a more extensive discussion about estrogen replacement therapy see Chapter 4.)

Sexuality

One of the myths about aging in our society says that older people are not and should not be sexually active and that there is something wrong with those who are. We know that this notion is false. Many studies and surveys have shown that older people can and do have satisfying sexual lives and that they maintain sexual functioning throughout their lifetimes.

Sexual interest and activity in older people usually continue the patterns set at an earlier stage of life. People who have enjoyed sexual activity throughout their lives continue to do so when they are older. However, people who were bored or un-interested in these activities earlier in life are not likely to change.

The physical ability to obtain sexual satisfaction remains intact throughout life. What does happen is that it may take a bit longer to become physically aroused. Vaginal lubrication and penile erection may take minutes rather than seconds. However, both men and women continue to have orgasms and to find sexual activity enjoyable and fulfilling. (For a fuller discussion of sexuality see Chapter 5.)

Intellectual Competence

Another myth about growing older is that we become "senile." In fact, the large majority of older people maintain intellectual and social competence and continue to function productively and normally throughout their lives. Occasional forgetfulness or confusion is not senility. Often these occur because of a temporary overload of information in the brain. This is understandable, since the older we are the more information we have accumulated and stored in our heads.

However, the myth persists, in part because many treatable illnesses can be, and are, misdiagnosed as senility. For example, people who are depressed or who are having a reaction to medication often appear confused, forgetful, or disorganized. They may be unable to care for themselves. In older people symptoms of readily recognized illnesses may be absent or may be different from the symptoms of younger people. If the health care practitioner is not aware of this, he or she may diagnose a physical illness as serious mental deterioration. The tragedy is that many people are incorrectly labeled as senile when their condition is actually treatable or even curable. (For additional information on causes and treatment of senility see Chapter 4.)

HEALTHY LIVING

We have a right to good health. This means we have the right to knowledge, as well as access to expert advice and treatment, which enable us to obtain the best health we can. But then it's up to us. No one can force us to be healthy. We have the responsibility to apply our newly gained knowledge to promote a healthy or healthier life style for ourselves.

This is the part of healthful living which is often difficult. After all, bad habits, even when we know they are unhealthy, are often very hard to break. However, the rewards are great, too. Who doesn't want to feel better, sleep better, be more relaxed, and live longer?

Exercise

We all know that we should exercise. However, many of us have been too busy, or felt inadequate or embarrassed, or didn't enjoy exercising and lost interest, or couldn't be bothered. At one time it was considered unfeminine to be sweaty. Worse, strenuous exercise was thought to be harmful to women.

In the 1970s these attitudes changed. People began to focus inward, and as they did, self-improvement, both physical and emotional, became a major goal. As both men and women recognized the relationship between physical fitness and better health, the various media took up the cause. We were bombarded with new ways to lose weight, exercise routines to be done during lunch hour, and the benefits of various sports activities. For women, this sudden access to a seemingly endless variety of exercise programs and sports was a revelation. Many of us realized for the first time that our bodies were capable of amazing things. Athletic grace and competence were not only a man's prerogatives. We discovered the ability to control and discipline our own bodies. This accomplishment has enhanced many a woman's self-image.

Obviously, regular exercise is not the answer to all life's problems but we can transfer the confidence which physical accomplishment provides to other facets of our lives. We see ourselves as "doers" rather than passive people to whom things happen. We become more actively involved in *how* we are living rather than merely existing. When we exercise regularly, we feel better about ourselves and, in turn, our positive outlook improves our physical health.

BENEFITS OF EXERCISE:

A regular exercise program has many benefits. It can:

1. Improve muscle tone.

2. Strengthen the heart.
3. Increase the circulation of blood throughout the body.
4. Provide a general sense of well-being.
5. Increase stamina.
6. Improve coordination.
7. Decrease chronic fatigue.
8. Work off tension.
9. Enhance the absorption and utilization of calcium in the body which, in turn, maintains strong bones (especially important to prevent osteoporosis).
10. Improve digestion.
11. Enhance sleep.
12. Aid in weight control.
13. Possibly decrease cholesterol and triglyceride levels in the blood.
14. Improve posture.

And, by doing all the above, exercise may retard aging.

TYPES OF EXERCISE:

Exercises can generally be divided into four different types, depending on how they affect the body. These are "aerobic," "anaerobic," "isotonic," and "isometric."

Aerobic exercises are vigorous movements which strengthen the heart and lungs by improving the processing of oxygen in the body. They involve continuous activity over a period of time. Examples of such exercises are brisk walking, jogging, swimming, and biking.

Anaerobic exercises are those which require short periods of intense activity which put a sudden high demand on the heart and lungs. These are "stop-and-start" exercises such as tennis.

Isotonic exercises are those which improve muscle strength and flexibility by putting these muscles through their complete range of motion. Examples are calisthenics and yoga.

Isometric exercises build muscle strength without movement by forcing muscles to work against each other or against immovable objects. Attempting to push over an immovable brick wall is an example. These exercises may be dangerous for older people, causing dizziness and fainting especially for those with high blood pressure. Isometric exercises are not recommended for older people by most health professionals.

The best exercise program for most older women (and men) is a combination of aerobic and isotonic exercises. A good program might be a brisk two-mile walk preceded and followed by several minutes of stretching and bending exercises. The stretching exercises double as warm-up and cool-down exercises performed for several minutes before or after the more strenuous activity.

TIPS ON PLANNING A SUCCESSFUL EXERCISE
PROGRAM:

1. Check with your health care practitioner before starting any exercise program. If you have not recently had a checkup, you will need a thorough physical examination and an electrocardiogram. A stress test (a special test in which an electrocardiogram monitors your heart as you run on a treadmill) may also be necessary.

2. Discuss your planned exercise program with your health care practitioner. Certain exercises or sports activities may not be recommended if you have a particular illness or medical condition.

3. Enjoy the activity you choose. You are more apt to continue a program if you are having fun.

4. Start slowly. No one can expect to run a marathon without preparation! Listen to your body. Don't push yourself to exhaustion. Doing a little bit more each time will build endurance gradually.

5. Do not start or stop exercising abruptly. A series of stretching exercises before and after more vigorous activity will prevent muscle tightening, increase flexibility, and prevent injury.

6. To gain the maximum effect, an exercise program should be performed for approximately thirty minutes three to five times a week. Starting slowly, work gradually up to this

goal over a period of week or months.

7. If you have trouble enjoying yourself, exercise with a friend. Companionship is a good incentive.

8. Exercise at your own pace—you don't have to compete with anyone.

9. Many women enjoy the exercise programs offered by the YWCA, YWHA, and other health clubs. These organizations often have qualified exercise instructors who plan individualized programs. Working out with an organized group provides support and encouragement. But membership can be expensive. You should try the facilities several times, if possible, before joining. Also, be sure to inquire about the refund policy in the event that you later decide to cancel your membership.

10. Wear comfortable, loose-fitting clothes. Cotton is usually most comfortable because it absorbs perspiration. In colder weather dress in several light layers rather than one heavy or bulky garment. Shoes should fit well and be appropriate for the activity you choose. If foot problems make fitting difficult, a podiatrist can prescribe the appropriate shoes, lifts, arch supports, or other aids.

EXERCISE MYTHS:

1. *Exercise increases the appetite.* Moderate exercise actually depresses the appetite and aids in weight control.

2. *Exercise is very tiring.* By increasing the circulation of blood throughout the body and by bringing oxygen to the tissues moderate exercise makes you more alert. As you become more fit, you will find you have more energy to get on with living.

3. *Exercise is not good for weight loss.* An exercise program will not result in a quick, dramatic weight loss. However, exercise activity does burn up calories. Therefore, over a period of time an exercise program will result in some weight loss even if you do not decrease your food intake. For example, a brisk three-mile walk four times a week should result in a thirteen-pound loss in one year without any reduction in food intake. Of course, an exercise program combined with a reduced-calorie diet will result in greater weight loss over the same period of time.

4. *"I am too old to exercise."* You are never too old to improve your physical condition. The health benefits are too great to ignore.

5. *"I get plenty of exercise in my daily activities; I don't need a planned program."* While maintaining an active life style is certainly beneficial to psychological health and well being, any exercise obtained is usually haphazard. One builds stamina, flexibility, endurance, and energy level by repeating the same movements or sports activities regularly. The trick is to incorporate them into your daily work. Do exercises for your fingers while washing

the dishes. Stretching and bending exercises can be done while putting away groceries or laundry. Possibilities are endless if you keep your mind on them.

Medications

Many older people use medications extensively and frequently. Eleven percent of the population of the United States is over 65, yet this age group takes about 25 percent of all prescription and over-the-counter drugs. (Over-the-counter medications are those purchased without a prescription such as aspirin, vitamins, laxatives, cold remedies, etc.) Eighty-five percent of older people take at least one prescription drug; the average older person fills thirteen prescriptions a year. Women generally take more medications than do men.

Medications can be lifesaving. They can control or cure many illnesses and relieve pain. However, they may also have serious side effects. In addition, aging changes often affect the way medication is absorbed, used and eventually eliminated from the body. There apparently are differences in the way women and men react to certain drugs. Older people may experience different side effects from medications than do young people, and may also require a smaller dose.

The effectiveness of some medications can be altered by alcohol, food, or other medications. For example, some antibiotics are not well absorbed into the bloodstream if they are taken with meals. Alcohol, combined with antihistamines, can lead to extreme drowsiness.

Finally, medications are very expensive. So, to spend money wisely, it is important to be well informed about the medications we take.

MEDICATION GUIDELINES:

1. Do not expect medication to be prescribed for every ailment or problem. In some cases medication is neither necessary nor desirable. There is no "magic pill" which cures everything.

2. If you do take medication, be sure you know:

   a) the name of each medication you take

   b) the reason you take the medication and how it affects your body (e.g., lower blood pressure, makes heart pump more efficiently)

   c) when and how often the medication should be taken (before, with, or after meals? only when symptoms occur? during the night as well as during waking hours? how many days should the medication be taken?)

   d) whether alcohol, food, or other medications affect the drug

   e) how the medication should be stored (in a dark place? is refrigeration necessary?)

3. If your health care practitioner does not provide information about medications, ask! The pharmacist may also be helpful.

4. Read the label and follow the instructions carefully. Do not take more than the recommended dosage.

5. Keep your health care practitioner informed of all medications you take, including over-the-counter drugs such as antacids, aspirin, and laxatives. You should also report any allergic reaction to a medication which you may have suffered in the past.

6. Long-term use of certain medications may affect your body's nutritional needs. For example, one type of diuretic or "water pill" used to treat high blood pressure or heart disease can cause the body to lose potassium. This loss can usually be replaced by eating foods high in potassium like oranges, raisins, and bananas. Again, it is important to check with your health care practitioner to see if this applies to you.

7. To save money ask your health care practitioner to prescribe a medication under its generic or chemical name rather than the brand name. Many medications are available this way, often at about half the price of the heavily advertised brand. There is usually no difference in quality, only in price. Comparison shopping is another way to save money, since prices may vary substantially at different pharmacies for the *same* medication.

8. Do not take medications prescribed for someone else or share your medications with others.

9. Do not save old medications. Most lose their effectiveness after a period of time; others become toxic. Many medications now carry an expiration date after which they should be discarded.

10. Alcohol is present in medications such as cough syrups, elixirs, and vitamin tonics. Caffeine is combined with aspirin in a number of pain relievers. If you have been told to avoid alcohol or caffeine, be sure to check the ingredients on the label of any medication you take.

OVER-THE-COUNTER-DRUGS:

These medications, which you can purchase without a prescription, are not necessarily harmless. Aspirin can cause stomach irritation and affect blood clotting; cold remedies can cause severe drowsiness. Over-the-counter drugs should be treated with the same seriousness that prescription drugs are. You should know the name and effect of the medication and follow instructions about dosage and precautions. Check labels for ingredients, especially if you have any allergies or if you must avoid alcohol or caffeine. Keep your health care practitioner informed of the over-the-counter drugs that you take, since they may interfere with the effectiveness of prescription medications.

Be aware of advertising gimmicks such as "special ingredients" or "extra strength." "Extra-strength" arthritis pain reliever may actually consist of one and a half aspirins at several times the price of aspirin. Read the labels.

Buy the most inexpensive version of the medication you need. The United States government sets standards for the chemical composition of all medications which manufacturers must meet. A drugstore's own brand of aspirin or aspirin substitute will usually be just as effective as the more expensive name brand.

Nutrition

The relationship between good nutrition and good health cannot be overemphasized. What we eat affects our overall well-being, including all our bodily functions, our energy level, our stamina, and our appearance. Good nutrition plays an important part in the prevention of some illnesses and is an essential part of the treatment in many others. We now know that eating habits play a role in such major health problems as high blood pressure, heart disease, and some types of cancer.

Unfortunately, many of us, for a variety of reasons, do not pay as much attention to our food choices as we should. Some of us think that there is no point in changing a lifetime of bad eating habits now. However, good nutrition can make us look and feel better and enable us to cope better with the rigors of daily living and to deal more successfully with short-term or chronic illnesses. Good nutrition is something we *can* do for ourselves.

AGING AND NUTRITION:

A number of aging changes may affect our food intake and eating habits. The first of these is a decrease in lean body mass, the amount of muscle we have in our bodies. Instead, we have a higher percentage of fat, which requires fewer calories for metabolism. Body fat is a very efficient user of calories. The net result is that we need fewer calories to maintain our weight. If we maintain or increase our caloric intake over the years, particularly if we have decreased our physical activities, we will gain weight. So, many of us must achieve good nutrition with fewer calories in order to maintain our body weight.

Another change is the reduced sense of taste and smell experienced by some older people. Obviously, this can affect appetite as well as the desire to eat certain types of food. Food intake and choices are affected if one has no teeth or if teeth are in poor condition. Dentures may interfere with taste sensation; ill-fitting ones may curb the consumption of hard or chewy foods. A decrease in muscle tone in the stomach and intestines slows down the passage of food and waste products and thus contributes to constipation.

In addition to these physical changes, older people have more such chronic illnesses as heart disease, high blood pressure, and diabetes, which require special dietary changes as part of treatment.

OTHER FACTORS AFFECTING NUTRITION:

Other factors beside physical changes affect nutrition in older people. The eating habits and cooking techniques of a lifetime affect what we eat and how we prepare it. We often continue to favor the foods of our ethnic heritage even when these are high in sodium, fat, and calories. Our religious beliefs may also affect our choice of foods.

Our physical and mental health influences what and how we eat. We have already mentioned a number of illnesses which require dietary modifications. If we are depressed, we may lose interest in food; conversely, some of us eat everything in sight when we feel sad. Some of us are nervous eaters, and anxiety keeps us nibbling compulsively. Others lose all interest in food during times of stress. The medications we take may affect our body's needs for certain nutrients, or we may have to avoid some types of food while taking a medication.

A sedentary life changes appetites. For some, a decrease in physical activity results in a corresponding decrease in appetite. For others, more free time means more snack time.

If mealtimes have usually been pleasant family or social occasions, eating may give us great pleasure. Food can symbolize security and safety. If, however, mealtimes have been associated with family friction or other unpleasantness, eating becomes a chore to complete as quickly as possible. Being alone and cooking for one can affect both choice and preparation of foods. The lack of eating companions may encourage us to skip meals altogether or to rely on convenience foods.

Obviously, financial limitations affect food

choices. Eating on a budget requires careful planning. In addition, food shopping and preparation may be difficult owing to a disabling illness, vagaries of the weather, or neighborhood safety.

WEIGHT:

Many of us have noticed the tendency to gain a few pounds over the years. Weight gain results from a combination of factors. It occurs simply because we take in more calories than we use up in energy. The excess stays in our bodies as fat. Our sedentary habits contribute to weight gain. With more time on our hands, many of us become constant "snackers" and actually increase instead of decrease the amount of food we eat. Also, some illnesses may limit our choice of foods, making it difficult to plan nutritious low-calories meals.

Our weight at age 25 can be an indicator of what we should weigh now. If it was "normal," we should maintain approximately that weight throughout our lives, since weight gain after that time usually consists of unneeded fat.

Another guide is the weight charts most often published in insurance companies' actuarial tables. They usually give a range of appropriate weight for height and bone structure.

Neither of these indicators takes into account the amount of body fat, however. A more accurate determination of appropriate weight is made by using a caliper to measure the percentage of body fat by measuring a skin fold. (A caliper is a measuring instrument used by some health care practitioners.)

By using this measurement, a well-muscled athlete with low percentage of body fat would not be considered overweight even though his weight is beyond weight chart range, whereas a sedentary person of the same weight with a high percentge of body fat would be considered too heavy.

Most of us know what weight is most appropriate for us and when we should lose weight. However, some of us are obsessed with thinness (in a society similarly obsessed), setting unrealistic weight goals for ourselves and then starving ourselves to attain them. Bodies come in all shapes and sizes. It is healthier to eat nutritionally balanced meals to maintain a weight at which we are comfortable than fast to become impossibly thin.

WEIGHT AND ILLNESS:

Recent studies have indicated that life expectancy is increased among those whose weight is normal or slightly above normal. Life expectancy was shorter among those either substantially underweight or overweight. Overweight people are at greater risk of developing diabetes, heart disease, high blood pressure, gall bladder disease, and several other illnesses. Overweight can also make osteoarthritis symptoms more severe by putting additional stress on affected joints. (For a more thorough discussion of overweight and obesity see Chapter 4.)

NUTRITIONAL REQUIREMENTS FOR OLDER WOMEN:

Good nutrition consists of following a sound,

healthy diet for life. (Diet, as used here, does not refer to weight loss but merely to the food that you eat every day.) A healthy diet provides all the essential nutrients: protein, carbohydrates, fat, vitamins, minerals, and water. We need these nutrients for energy (calories), to build, maintain, and repair body tissues; and to regulate body processes.

We obtain these necessary nutrients from the four basic food groups.

Milk Group—Items: milk, cheese, yogurt, cottage cheese, ice cream, buttermilk.
Provides: protein, calcium, riboflavin (vitamin B_2), fat, phosphorus.
2 servings daily.
1 serving = 1 cup of milk (whole, skim, lowfat, buttermilk)
1 cup of yogurt
1 ½ ounces of cheddar cheese
1 ½ cups of cottage cheese
1 ¾ cups of ice cream

Note: To prevent osteoporosis, many experts recommend increasing milk group servings to 3–4 per day. (See section on calcium later in this chapter for more information on other sources of calcium.)

½ cup of evaporated milk + ½ cup of water = 1 cup of milk. 1 cup of reconstituted dry milk = 1 cup of fluid milk.
Skim (nonfat) milk and low-fat (99%) milk are

lower in calories and fat than regular (whole) milk.

Skim milk = 90 calories/8 ounces

Low-fat milk = 110 calories/8 ounces

Whole milk = 165 calories/8 ounces

Powdered dry milk is a low-cost alternative to fluid milk. If taste is a problem, ½ cup of reconstituted powdered milk can be mixed with ½ cup of fluid milk.

Meat Group—Items: meat, fish, poultry, eggs, dry beans or peas, peanut butter.

Provides: protein, fat, iron, thiamine (B_1), niacin, zinc, phosphorus.

2 servings daily.

1 serving = 2 ounces of cooked lean meat, fish, poultry

2 eggs

1 cup of cooked dry beans, peas, or lentils

4 tablespoons of peanut butter

¾ cup of soybean curd (tofu)

⅓ cup of nuts or seeds (pumpkin, sesame, sunflower, etc.)

Prepared luncheon meats, sausages and peanut butter are high in undesirable sodium and fat.

Fruit and Vegetable Group—Items: all vegetables and fruits.

Provides: Vitamin A, vitamin C, carbohydrates, fiber.

4 servings daily. 1 serving should be a fruit or vegetable rich in vitamin C. A fruit or vegetable

rich in vitamin A should be included 3–4 times per week.

1 serving = 1 cup of raw fruit or vegetable
  ½ cup of juice
  ½ cup of cooked fruit or vegetable
  ½ cup of canned fruit
  1 medium-sized apple, peach, orange, banana, potato, etc.
  ½ medium-sized grapefruit
  1 wedge melon

Food rich in vitamin C are citrus fruits and juices (oranges, lemons, grapefruit), cantaloupe, strawberries, papaya, broccoli, green peppers, potatoes cooked in their skins, tomatoes, tomato juice.

Foods rich in vitamin A are orange or dark green leafy vegetables such as carrots, cantaloupe, squash, apricots, pumpkin, spinach, chard, kale, watercress, turnip greens.

Fresh fruits and vegetables usually taste best but are often the most expensive unless bought in season.

Frozen vegetables and fruits provide the same nutrients as fresh and are usually cheaper. For example, there is no difference in nutrient value between a glass of frozen orange juice and a glass of freshly squeezed juice.

Most canned vegetables are high in sodium since sodium is added during packing. Most canned fruits are packed in sugar syrup which adds unnecessary sugar and calories to the fruit. (Check labels for ingredients.) Water-packed and low sodium canned fruits and vegetables are available, but usually at a higher price than regular canned goods.

Bread, Cereal, and Grain Group—Items: enriched, or whole grain breads and spaghetti, macaroni, and other pasta; cornmeal, rolled oats, flour, grits, crackers.
    Provides: carbohydrates, protein, iron, B vitamins, fiber.
    4 servings daily.
    1 serving = 1 slice of bread
                  1 cup of ready-to-eat cereal
                  ½ cup of cooked cereal, pasta, rice, grits, noodles.
                  2 graham crackers
                  1 small biscuit or muffin

Whole grain breads and cereals are recommended because the refining process removes most of the B vitamins, vitamin E, fiber, and minerals. Enriched flour is refined flour to which three of the B vitamins lost in processing have been replaced.

Whole grain products can be a cheap, filling, and nourishing source of protein when combined with a small amount of animal protein. Examples are cereal with milk, macaroni and cheese.

Baked goods such as pies, cakes, and cookies are usually made with refined white flour and are high in sugar, fat, and sodium. Commercially baked goods, in addition, often have preservatives, stabilizers, and artificial ingredients added. If used at all, these foods should be taken in limited amounts.

Check labels! Some "natural" whole grain cereals, such as some granolas, are high in fat, calories, and added sugar, and are very expensive.

Most people use some foods not listed in the four major food groups to round out their meals and to meet energy needs. These include fats such as butter, margarine, vegetable oils, lard, salad dressing, cream, and cream cheese. Although fats are a concentrated source of energy, they provide more calories per gram than either protein or carbohydrates and should be used in limited amounts.

Desserts and sweets such as cakes, pies, cookies, ice cream, candy, and chocolate are high in calories, sugar, and fat and are low in other nutrients. With caloric needs as well as budgets limited, it is healthier to cut down the amount of "empty" calories we consume. The best desserts and snacks are fruits and vegetables, which are high in nutrients and relatively low in calories. If you must eat dessert, concentrate on those made with milk, milk products, or whole grain with a limited amount of sugar.

WATER:
Water is not really a nutrient; however, it is more important to life than food is. It makes up more than 60 percent of the body and is crucial to many body functions. Water carries nutrients and removes waste products; regulates body temperature; and is necessary for digestion, absorption, excretion, and circulation. It helps prevent constipation by aiding peristalsis.

The daily requirement is at least six glasses of water a day. Although water can be obtained from food (fruits and vegetables have a high percentage of water) and other liquids such as soups and juices, water alone is refreshing, healthy, and has no calories. (Coffee and tea are not good substitutes, since both contain caffeine and other irritants.)

SAMPLE DAILY MEAL PLAN USING THE FOUR BASIC FOOD GROUPS:

Breakfast	*Example*
Fruit/Vegetable Group—1 serving (vitamin C rich)	1 orange
Milk Group—1 serving	Milk—1 glass
Meat Group—½ serving	Egg
Grain Group—1–2 servings	Shredded wheat, bran muffin, or whole wheat bread
Beverage (optional)	Coffee or tea

Lunch	
Meat Group—½—1 serving	Open-faced tuna salad sandwich on whole wheat bread (1 slice)
Grain Group—1 serving	
Fruit/Vegetable Group—1 serving	Sliced tomatoes and lettuce
Milk Group—1 serving	Vanilla pudding made with milk

Beverage (optional)	Apple cider—1 glass

Dinner

Meat Group—1 serving	Beef stew
Fruit/Vegetable Group—2 or 3 servings	Small baked potato, steamed broccoli, baked pear
Grain Group—1–2 servings	Dinner roll
Beverage (optional)	

This is only a sample to illustrate how balanced meals are planned. For example, you may vary your diet by having your biggest meal at lunch instead of at dinner, saving a grain group serving for a snack, eating two slices of toast at breakfast, and so on. You may want to divide three meals into five or six smaller meals. Also, standard servings of all the foods listed may result in weight loss or weight gain depending on energy needs and exercise and may have to be adjusted to suit your own needs. If you adjust, make sure that you include some portion of all the food groups mentioned.*

Calories are energy supplied by food. If you take in more food than your body can use in energy, it is stored as fat and you will gain weight. If you eat less food than your body requires in energy, you will lose weight. If you are at your correct weight

*This sample plan is based on the needs of older women in reasonably good health. Diet modifications may have to be made because of illness—heart disease, high blood pressure, diabetes, or after surgery.

and are maintaining that weight, your food/caloric intake is adequate in amount consumed. The recommended ranges for women are:

Age 23–50—1600–2400 calories/day
Age 51–75—1400–2200 calories/day
Age 76+ —1200–2000 calories/day

An area of controversy concerning our daily food intake is the proportion of calories we allot to the three basic energy sources: protein, fat, and carbohydrates. The average American diet is now approximately:

42% fat
12% protein
46% carbohydrates

This high-fat diet has been linked to a number of illnesses, including heart disease and breast and colon cancer. Experts in nutrition now recommend a change in diet composition to one which is:

30% fat (a decrease in fat)
12% protein (no change)
58% carbohydrates (an increase in carbohydrates, especially complex carbohydrates such as whole grains, and dried peas and beans)

The most widely used source for nutritional and caloric requirements is the table of Recommended Dietary Allowances (RDA) developed by the Food and Nutrition Board of the National Academy of Sciences. The RDAs, most recently revised in 1980, indicate the levels of essential nutrients and calories necessary for various groups of people. Since they are standards which cover both a variety of groups and nutritional needs, the values listed *exceed* the requirements of most healthy people and are not intended to be used to evaluate individual diets. In addition, the RDA makes no specific recommendations for older people except for caloric needs. Otherwise, all older people are lumped into the age category 51 + . (This reflects the deplorable lack of research into the nutritional requrements of those over 65.) However, the RDA can be useful as a *guide* to meal planning and is the basis for the recommended daily servings of the four basic food groups.

The Department of Health and Human Services recently (1980) published a list of recommendations called *Dietary Guidelines for Americans*. These are:

1. Eat a variety of foods.
2. Maintain ideal weight.
3. Avoid too much fat, saturated fat, and cholesterol.
4. Eat foods with adequate starch and fiber.
5. Avoid too much sugar.
6. Avoid too much sodium.
7. If you drink alcohol, do so in moderation.

All easier said than done! However, by being informed consumers we can learn to develop nutritious eating habits.

1. *It is important to eat a variety of foods* in order to obtain all the necessary nutrients. No one food is "perfect," and anyway it is boring to eat the same thing all the time. Variety stimulates the appetite and is a pleasant way to get all the nutrients you need.

2. *Fresh, canned, and frozen foods* all have advantages and disadvantages. Fresh foods taste better and are usually lower in calories. However, they are perishable. Canned or frozen foods are usually cheaper and less perishable than are fresh foods. They come in convenient sizes and can be stored for longer periods of time. Taste and texture are often altered, however. The calorie count will be higher if the food contains added sugar, starch, fat, or sauce. In addition, salt and other sodium compounds, artificial colors or flavorings, stabilizers, and preservatives such as BHA or nitrates and nitrites (in cured meats) may have been added. Check labels before you buy.

3. So-called *convenience foods* (e.g., frozen dinners; canned pasta with sauce; "fast foods" such as hamburgers, hot dogs, and pizza) are usually more expensive per serving than those made from scratch but do save preparation time for busy people. However, these and other processed foods may have added

salt, sugar, preservatives, and artificial ingredients, and they are usually high in fat as well. The consumer must weigh convenience and time saved against cost and nutritional value to make an informed choice.

4. Develop the habit of *reading labels*. Most canned and packaged foods must have the ingredients listed on the label. They are listed in order of prevalence; that is, the first ingredient listed is present in the largest amount, the next ingredient is second largest, and so on. For example, the better buy in tomato sauces is the one which lists tomatoes rather than water as the first ingredient. Additives such as salt, preservatives, coloring, and flavoring are also listed.

   Other nutritional information may also be available on a label. Some foods list calories per serving, the amount of certain nutrients present (e.g., protein, fat, and carbohydrates), and the percentage of the Recommended Dietary Allowance (RDA) for such nutrients.

5. If you take *medications*, check with your health care practitioner to ascertain when medication should be taken (before, with, or after meals; with water, milk, or juice) and whether any foods should be avoided.

6. Prepare food to conserve nutrients. Do not overcook vegetables or fruit. Better yet, eat them steamed or raw. If you must cook vegetables in water, use as little as possible and

do not discard it. Use it in soups, stews, or broth.

7. Be aware of *food fads*. There are no magic foods, vitamins, food supplements, or tonics which will cure all your ills. A diet based solely on one food such as eggs or grapefruit is not balanced and will not provide all needed nutrients. Most fads are unhealthy *and* expensive.

8. *"Health foods"* have become an important part of the food industry in the past decade. Many consumers, tired of bland, overprocessed, expensive food and food products, are worried about additives, preservatives and chemical fertilizers. They want food which, instead of being processed, has been kept in its natural state. Health foods have thus become big business. Many health food stores have high prices and use sophisticated marketing and packaging techniques to lure customers into purchasing items which may not even be healthy. Anything which is called a "health food" or "all natural" is not necessarily nutritious. For example, "natural" potato chips and candy bars are high in natural fat, sugar, sodium, and calories but supply little in the way of other nutrients. Many whole grain cereals are loaded with sugar, a "natural" ingredient, making them substantially higher in calories than some commercially prepared non-health-food cereals. It is just as important to read ingredi-

ent labels on foods labeled "natural" or "all natural" as on any others. Because a food lacks preservatives or chemical additives does not necessarily mean that it is good for you.

Cost and taste are other important considerations in selecting "health foods." Such foods as whole grain breads and cereals, whole grain flours, and dried fruits have been available in supermarkets and grocery stores for years at lower prices. With the benefit of fancy packaging and "health food" status they now sell for higher prices in health food or specialty stores. Once again— be an informed consumer: read labels, compare prices, and be skeptical of gimmicks and miracle claims.

9. *Artificial sweetners* such as saccarin, aspartame, and cyclamates are chemical compounds used as sugar substitutes because they taste sweet. They have fewer calories than sugar, since they cannot be metabolized by the body. Saccharin and aspartane are the only artificial sweeteners in current use. Both saccharin and cyclamates (which were banned in this country in 1969) have been reported in various studies to cause several types of cancer in laboratory animals. While this link to cancer has not been proven in humans, the possibility is there. Some recent studies suggest that aspartane can affect chemical reactions in the brain, causing a va-

riety of symptoms such as headaches and depression. Until we have more definitive evidence, the prudent course would seem to be to limit the amount of artificial sweeteners we consume or to avoid them altogether. (Diabetics who use artificial sweeteners should follow the advice of their health care practitioner.) Artificial sweeteners are found in low-calorie or "diet" soft drinks and in many foods labeled "dietetic" or "low calorie." Check labels for content information.

10. *Food additives* worry many people. Additives range from the most common, sugar, to spices, herbs, natural and artificial flavors, salt, vitamins, and minerals. They also include artificial colors, emulsifiers, and stabilizers which maintain texture; antioxidants such as BHA which prevent rancidity; and nitrates and nitrites which prevent botulism in cured meats. Most food additives were originally intended to enhance flavor or color, provide a uniform product, or protect the consumer from illness. However, some additives are themselves increasingly being linked to disease. For example, sugar provides little more than extra calories, and salt is linked to high blood pressure. Some food coloring and preservatives have been linked to various cancers in animals.

11. *Food marketing and storage*
    a) Make a grocery list before you food-shop. Don't shop when you are hungry

or tired. Note items you already have on hand and try to plan meals around them as well as around leftovers which must be used. You'll cut down on impulse buying and keep within your food budget.

b) Watch for, and take advantage of, specials. You may also want to use "cents-off" coupons, but compare prices before you buy. Often another brand or the store's own brand is cheaper than buying with a coupon.

c) Many stores now offer what are called "generic foods" packaged in plain containers at prices even lower than the store's brands. These are items such as canned fruit or vegetables which are a grade or two below "Fancy" or "Choice" but which contain the same nutrients as their more expensive counterparts. They have been welcomed by many consumers to whom price is more important than appearance.

d) Read labels and check ingredients before you buy. This is particularly important if you must follow a special diet or avoid certain foods.

e) Compare prices before you buy. Name-brand products are more expensive than store brands and may be no better in quality.

f) Supermarkets are usually cheaper and offer greater variety than small grocery stores. However, getting to them can require a long walk or trip on public transportation—worth considering if you must carry several bags or push home a heavy shopping cart. Small grocery stores, while usually more expensive, may be more convenient and may extend credit, cash checks, and offer free delivery.

g) Try to keep basic foods and a few staples on hand which can be used to make nutritious meals if you are unable to food-shop because of illness or bad weather. Powdered milk; flour; peanut butter; and dried fruit such as raisins and prunes, and canned fruits, vegetables, soups, and tuna fish are good examples. However, you do not need enough food to feed an army. Overstocking is expensive and wasteful.

h) Bags of frozen vegetables are a good buy because they can be opened to obtain amounts needed, with the balance kept frozen. A loaf of bread can be sliced and frozen. Individual slices thaw quickly, and there is no waste. Day-old bread is cheaper than fresh bread. Cereals which must be cooked are cheaper than instant or ready-to-eat cereals.

i) If you live alone or with one other person, you may find it more practical to purchase the medium or small size of an item which can then be used within a reasonable length of time. It is not economical to buy the large size, only to discard part of it when it isn't used. If a large purchase is a particularly good buy (such as twenty pounds of potatoes or a fifteen-pound turkey), consider sharing the produce, cost, and savings with neighbors or friends.

j) Those on a limited budget may be eligible for the federal government's food stamp program. Food stamps can help stretch tight budgets, and you need not be on welfare or public assistance to qualify for them.

k) If you *live alone*, try to share a meal with a friend on a regular basis. You can split costs or take turns in planning and preparation. Either way, companionship makes mealtime more pleasant.

Nutrition Pluses and Minuses

PROTEIN:

Proteins are the body's building blocks. They are used for growth, maintenance, and repair of body cells, and in the production of enzymes and hormones. They are a very important part of our diets and should constitute 12 percent of our daily caloric intake.

To many people, protein has the image of being the best, the healthiest, and the most important nutrient, which in turn is interpreted as "the more, the better." Carbohydrates and starchy foods, on the other hand, are seen as foods which are not as healthy as protein and which are likely to make an individual gain weight. Consequently, many people eat much more protein than they need while eliminating valuable carbohydrates and starches from their daily food intake. In doing so, they concentrate on eating animal protein (meat, cheese, dairy products) which tend to be high in fat, calories, and cholesterol. Several research studies have shown that there is a link between a high-fat diet and heart disease and certain types of cancer. A better choice would be to increase the number of carbohydrate calories consumed (especially complex carbohydrates such as starchy vegetables and grains) while decreasing the amount of animal protein. Many people do not realize that complex carbohydrates contain protein, too, being composed of protein and carbohydrate instead of protein and fat as animal protein is. (Ounce for ounce, fat contains more than twice the number of calories of protein or carbohydrate.) It is a healthier way to eat.

On the other hand, some older women, especially those on tight food budgets, do not eat enough protein. Sources of animal protein such as meat, cheese, and fish are expensive. Milk, while comparatively inexpensive, is often not drunk out of the mistaken belief that adults do not need milk. Many do not realize that plant and grain proteins, when combined with each other or with small amounts of animal protein, are as nutritious as animal protein alone.

Proteins are made up of amino acids. Out of approximately twenty amino acids, nine are called essential. These must be obtained from food because they cannot be manufactured by the body. The other amino acids are necessary for body functions, but since they can be manufactuured by the body they are not essential in the diet.

Foods which contain all nine essential amino acids are referred to as complete protein foods. They are those proteins of animal origin—milk, meat, cheese, eggs—plus soybeans. Those foods which contain fewer than the nine essential amino acids are termed incomplete protein foods and are those of plant origin—grains, legumes, seeds, and nuts. However, these plant foods, when used together, can complement each other by providing all nine essential amino acids, thus becoming complete proteins. That is, one food can supply the amino acids which are lacking in the other, so that together they supply all nine essential amino acids. Examples are rice and beans, cornmeal and kidney beans (used in many Mexican foods), and peanut butter on whole grain bread. Plant protein can also be combined with a small amount of animal protein in foods such as macaroni and cheese, and cereal with milk. This is the way vegetarians get complex proteins into their diets. In fact, with its stress on whole grains and other complex carbohydrates, and the omission of meat from the diet, vegetarianism is closer to the daily diet most nutrition experts are recommending than the typical American diet is.

(Even those vegetarians who omit milk, eggs, and cheese from their diet in addition to meat can obtain enough protein and all essential amino acids from plant protein, but doing this takes very careful planning.) The point is that, whereas meat is a complete protein, you do not have to eat it every day, or at all, to be healthy, and meat substitutes are usually cheaper than meat.

CHOLESTEROL:

Cholesterol is an essential body compound needed to build cell membranes and to produce several hormones, bile acids, and vitamin D. The body can make all the cholesterol it needs on its own. However, cholesterol is also obtained in foods, mainly animal products, such as whole milk, meat, egg yolks, butter, cheese, organ meats, shrimp, and oysters. The average American diet is rich in these foods and therefore is high in cholesterol.

Many middle-aged and older Americans have an elevated blood cholesterol, a level above 200–220 mg. An elevated blood cholesterol has been found to be one of the three major risk factors for heart disease, along with cigarette smoking and high blood pressure. (Heart disease is the leading cause of death in the United States.) Cholesterol has been shown to be part of the fatty buildup called atherosclerosis which clogs arteries. Several studies have shown a very strong link between a diet high in cholesterol and atherosclerosis and heart disease.

In addition to the amount of cholesterol, the amount of fat in the diet must be taken into consideration. Fats are divided into two categories, saturated and unsaturated. Saturated fats tend to be the more solid, animal fats and are found in meat, fish, poultry, whole milk, cream, cheese, baked goods, and butter; they are also found in some vegetable oils such as coconut and palm oils, hydrogenated margarine, and cocoa. Unsaturated fats are found in liquid vegetable oils such as corn, safflower, and sesame oils and in unhydrogenated margarine. Saturated fats in the diet tend to raise the blood cholesterol level. Since the typical American diet is over 40 percent fat, the type of fat eaten is an important factor affecting the blood cholesterol level. At this time, however, no one knows the long-term effects on the body of a high unsaturated-fat diet, and such a diet is not recommended.

No study can prove that a high-fat, high-cholesterol diet *causes* heart disease. (Such a study would take thousands of human volunteers many years and be a difficult and expensive undertaking.) However, many studies *have* shown that countries with high-fat, high-cholesterol diets, like the United States, have a high incidence of heart disease. In countries where the diet is low in both fats and cholesterol, the incidence of death from heart disease is correspondingly low (e.g., Japan). When Japanese people move to the United States and begin to eat as we do, their rates of heart disease also rise. Other studies have shown that blood cholesterol levels can be decreased by following a low-fat, low-cholesterol diet.

In view of this type of evidence, most nutrition

experts now recommend several dietary changes:

1. Decrease the amount of cholesterol in your diet. (Foods high in cholesterol include whole milk, cream, egg yolks, cheese, butter, red meat, organ meats, shrimp, and oysters.)
2. Decrease total fat consumption. (Foods high in fat include whole milk, cheese, meat, butter, baked goods, peanut butter, nuts, and processed foods.) Poultry, veal, and fish have less fat than beef and pork. Use skim milk or dried milk for drinking or cooking to decrease both cholesterol and fat in your diet.
3. Within the category of decreased fat consumption the amount of saturated fats should also be reduced. Instead, substitute unsaturated fats. For example, use vegetable oils or unhydrogenated margarine in place of butter or lard. (*Hydrogenated* margarine contains saturated fat, which gives it its firm consistency.) Decreasing overall fat consumption is also helpful to weight watchers, since fat has more than twice as many calories as do protein or carbohydrate.
4. Increase consumption of complex carbohydrates as a substitute for fats. They provide roughage (fiber) and are lower in calories than fat. There is also some evidence that they help lower blood cholesterol.
5. Maintain ideal weight. Overweight people have higher blood cholesterol levels than do those of normal weight.

FIBER:

Fiber is the indigestible part of plant foods—vegetables, fruits, grains, and nuts. It is also called roughage. There are a number of different types of fiber. For example, cellulose, which is insoluble in water, is found in bran and whole grains, while pectins and gums, which are water soluble, are present in a number of fruits and vegetables, dried beans, and oatmeal.

The American diet tends to be low in fiber and high in refined foods. In recent years the high-fiber diet has been cited as a prevention or cure for many diseases, ranging from gallstones to cancer. Although many of these claims have not been substantiated, a *moderate* amount of fiber is now thought to be an important part of a well-balanced diet and does have several healthful benefits. Of course, anyone with an intestinal illness should check with a health care practitioner before beginning self-treatment with fiber.

Constipation. Fiber helps to prevent constipation because it absorbs water, making the stool softer and larger while speeding up its passage through the bowel. Whole grain breads and cereals; old-fashioned oatmeal (not instant); raw, unpeeled fruits such as apples, pears, and berries; and root vegetables are most effective.

Although it is not necessary, many people use bran for this purpose, adding it to soups, cereals, muffins, pancakes, and other baked goods. If bran is used, several precautions should be taken. Bran should be added gradually to your diet. Start with as little as one teaspoon, working up gradually to two to three tablespoons per day. Drink plenty of fluids daily; otherwise the bran itself may cause constipation or stool impaction. Be sure to check labels; bran cereals are often sugared (adding extra calories) and expensive.

Large amounts of bran may cause intestinal gas and abdominal distention, may irritate the stomach and intestines, and may reduce the absorption of necessary nutrients.

Cholesterol. Recent research indicates that some dietary fiber helps reduce blood cholesterol levels. The effective fibers are the pectins and gums found in fruits, vegetables, oats, and beans. Bran (cellulose), however, is *not* effective. There is evidence of an association between cancer of the colon (the second most common type of cancer among both men and women) and a low-fiber diet. Dietary fiber is also thought to be useful in prevention and treatment of diverticula—outpouchings of the intestinal lining which may become inflamed and infected. At this time, there is at best only conflicting evidence as to the benefit of dietary fiber in other intestinal illnesses such as irritable bowel syndrome, colitis, or Crohn's disease (regional enteritis).

Fiber may be useful in lowering the blood sugar of diabetics and in preventing or controlling obesity by providing bulk in the diet to make us feel full.

To add more fiber to your diet:

1. Eat whole grain breads and cereals, brown rice, and raw fruits and vegetables with their

skins. (Processed and refined foods are low in fiber.)

2. Check labels to make sure that products contain whole grains—whole wheat, whole oats, etc.
3. Use whole grain cereals instead of bread crumbs in meat loaf and meatballs.
4. Snack on fruits and vegetables instead of on sweets.
5. Be sure to drink a generous amount of fluid each day—six or more glasses—especially water.

SODIUM:

Sodium, essential for proper cell functioning and the maintenance of water balance in the body, is present naturally in most foods and is added to many others. Americans consume approximately six to eight grams of sodium daily, over twice the estimated adequate and safe intake of one to three grams per day.

Much sodium intake, in the form of salt (sodium chloride), is added in cooking and at the table, and is present in many commercially prepared and processed foods. Our taste for so much salt is acquired; we need not add it to our food. There is enough natural sodium in food to provide the amount we need.

A high-sodium/salt diet increases the chance of developing high bood pressure, especially for those already at risk. High blood pressure, in turn, increases the risk of both heart attack and stroke.

Treatment for high blood pressure includes a low-sodium diet in addition to medication and weight loss, if necessary. If you have high blood pressure, you will need detailed instructions on dietary restrictions as well as lists of acceptable and unacceptable foods from your health care practitioner.

Because of concerns about salt, dietary experts have recommended that all people, including those in good health, reduce the amount of salt/sodium consumed. Following are some hints for healthy people who wish to cut down on their salt/sodium intake.

1. Use salt sparingly or not at all in cooking and at the table. Get into the habit of tasting food before automatically salting it.

2. Read labels on the food you buy. Many canned and processed foods have added salt (sodium chloride) or other sodium compounds such as monosodium glutamate (MSG), sodium benzoate, baking powder, baking soda, sodium nitrite, and sodium nitrate. Try to find similar foods without these additives.

3. Avoid obviously salty foods such as canned nuts, pretzels, potato chips, crackers, pickles, olives, and salted, smoked, or processed meats such as bacon, luncheon meat, sausage, ham, frankfurters, canned sardines, canned soups, broth, and bouillon.

4. Commercially prepared baked foods have added salt as well as baking soda and other

sodium compounds. Many breakfast cereals also have added sodium. Three which do not are puffed rice, puffed wheat, and shredded wheat. Check labels.

5. Other foods high in sodium are cheese (except unsalted cottage cheese and low-sodium cheeses which are specifically labeled as such), commercial salad dressings, ketchup, prepared mustard, soy sauce, Worcestershire sauce, meat tenderizers, and salted peanut butter.

6. Use unsalted butter or margarine.

7. Do not use garlic, onion, or celery salts as salt substitutes. These are merely table salt with flavoring added. There are commercially prepared salt substitutes made with potassium. These should be used only on the advice of your health care practitioner.

8. Experiment with herbs, spices, and other flavorings to take the place of salt. Fresh or dried basil, dill, rosemary, tarragon, and thyme, as well as cinnamon, cloves, peppers, onion, garlic, and lemon add interesting flavors to food.

9. Over-the-counter drugs may contain large amounts of salt. Check labels.

10. Check with your local water company to find out how much sodium the drinking water in your community contains. Water which is softened may contain large amounts of sodium.

11. Because of consumer demand, more com-

mercially prepared foods are being produced and marketed as "low-sodium" or "low-salt" foods. They are often very expensive, however. If you decide to buy these foods, *read labels and compare prices.*

CAFFEINE:

Caffeine, a substance present in several foods and medications, is ingested in substantial amounts by a great many people. Coffee is the major source of caffeine, but it is also present in tea, cocoa, chocolate, cola drinks, and some other types of soda as well as in a number of over-the-counter medications such as pain relievers (Anacin, Excedrin), cold remedies (Dristan), stimulants (No-Doz), weight-loss pills, and some prescription drugs. Medically, caffeine is classified as a drug because of the number of effects it has on the body. Though countless people use caffeine to wake them up and keep them alert during the day it can cause anxiety, restlessness, depression, irritability, upset stomach, sleep disturbances, increased heart and breathing rate, and irregular heartbeat and palpitations. It also raises blood pressure slightly and increases the amount of digestive juices present in the stomach. These effects may complicate such illnesses as heart disease, high blood pressure, depression, or ulcer. The effects of caffeine will depend on your tolerance and on how much you consume. Some people cannot tolerate even one cup of coffee per day; others drink six cups or more without noticing any bad effects.

The public worries more about the effects of caffeine because of recent studies showing a possible link between caffeine and cystic breast disease, caffeine and birth defects, and coffee and cancer of the pancreas. Many people find that they have developed a dependency on caffeine's stimulant effect, and without it they are listless, sluggish, sleepy, and irritable.

For most people, the amount of caffeine present in one to two cups of coffee per day poses no problem. (One cup of coffee contains approximately 100–150 mg of caffeine, depending on the strength of the brew. This compares with approximately 30–50 mg of caffeine in a cup of tea, 40 mg in a can of cola beverage, and 10 mg in a cup of cocoa.) However, those who are very sensitive to the effects of caffeine should avoid it entirely. If you have an illness which may be affected by caffeine (heart disease, high blood pressure, depression, ulcer), follow the advice of your health care practitioner. You may have to limit your caffeine intake or eliminate it.

DECAFFEINATED COFFEE AND CAFFEINE SUBSTITUTES:

There are beverages which can be substituted for caffeine-containing drinks. Decaffeinated coffee still contains a small amount of caffeine. Most commercial brands available are decaffeinated by being treated with methylene chloride, a chemical about which some questions of safety have been raised. However, most brands use this chemical in much smaller amounts than the maximum ruled safe by the Food and Drug Administration. Some expensive decaffeinated blends sold in specialty stores use water or steam to decaffeinate, thereby avoiding use of the chemical.

Decaffeinated coffee can be used for some or all of your regular coffee intake or mixed with regular coffee to provide coffee with a lower caffeine content. Grain-based beverages which contain no caffeine (Pero, Postum) can be used as substitutes. Although tea and cocoa both contain caffeine, they have less than coffee. Most herb teas do not contain caffeine, but check the ingredient label to be sure. Also read labels on soft drinks. Most colas and some other sodas do contain caffeine, although consumer pressure has resulted in the removal of caffeine from some soft drinks and the marketing of new no-caffeine sodas.

To avoid caffeine in over-the-counter medications, read labels on all medications. Some pain relievers, cold remedies, allergy tablets, stimulants, and diet pills contain caffeine.

CALCIUM:

Calcium is a mineral essential for the growth and maintenance of bones. It is also necessary for blood clotting, muscle contraction and relaxation, nerve impulse transmission, and cell and enzyme functioning. We store two to three pounds of calcium in our bodies—99 percent of it in the bones and teeth and the rest in the muscles and body fluids.

The body closely regulates the amount of calcium in the blood. If the level drops because of low dietary intake or certain illnesses, the necessary calcium will be transferred from the bones into the bloodstream. On the other hand, when the calcium level in the blood is adequate, any additional calcium is stored in the bones for future use.

Long-term deficiency of calcium in the diet is considered a contributing factor in the development of osteoporosis. In this illness, which occurs most often among older women, there is a decrease in the amount of bone in the body, possibly resulting in fractures with little or no obvious cause.

The recommended Dietary Allowance for older women is 800 mg of calcium per day, about the amount in three cups of milk. Some experts in the prevention and treatment of osteoporosis recommend a daily calcium intake equal to a quart of milk per day.

Other sources of calcium besides milk are yogurt, cottage cheese, hard cheese, sardines and salmon eaten with the bones, green leafy vegetables (except spinach), dried figs, egg yolks, and nuts. However, milk and milk products are the best sources of calcium, and it is hard to get enough calcium without them. Also, calcium is best obtained from food rather than from supplements or pills because it is most readily absorbed when eaten in small amounts throughout the day. If you cannot tolerate milk or milk products, check with your health care practitioner. You may have an enzyme (lactase) deficiency which prevents milk from being digested properly. This lack of tolerance can be overcome by using specially prepared milk to which the missing enzyme has been added, or by adding the enzyme to the milk yourself (a commercially prepared enzyme is available). Do not take calcium supplements without the advice of your health care practitioner.

Absorption of calcium in the body is enhanced when there are adequate amounts of vitamin C, vitamin D, and protein in the diet. Absorption is also increased by exercise. (That is why exercise builds strong bones!) Absorption is decreased by aging, medications such as steroids, oxalic and phytic acids found in spinach and legumes, and possibly by a high-fat, high-protein, high-phosphate diet. (Foods high in phosphorous are meat, soft drinks, and processed foods.) Some medications (such as aluminum-containing antacids) increase calcium loss in the urine.

Immobilization (as in a cast) or confinement to a bed or a wheelchair for long periods of time cause bone decalcification. This excess calcium must be excreted in the urine, which increases the risk of developing kidney stones. People thus restricted should maintain an adequate but not excessive calcium intake followed closely by the health care practitioner.

VITAMINS:

Vitamins are substances required by the body in small amounts to regulate a variety of functions in the cells. Contrary to what many people think, vitamins do not provide extra energy or pep. However, they must be included in the diet, since they are not produced in the body in sufficient amounts.

Vitamins are divided into two groups: fat-soluble

and water-soluble. The fat-soluble vitamins (A, D, E, K), which are stored in the body, are not easily excreted, so that excessive intake can be dangerous. On the other hand, the water-soluble vitamins (B complex, C), which are not stored in the body, are easily eliminated in the urine, and they must be obtained every day. High intake of water-soluble vitamins is less likely to cause problems, but undesirable effects have been reported, especially with vitamin C.

FAT-SOLUBLE VITAMINS

Vitamin A is necessary for healthy skin, teeth, and bones, and to produce the eye pigment which is needed to see in dim light. It is found in animal products such as fish-liver oils, liver, butter, cream, egg yolks, and in fortified skim milk and margarine. Carotene is a substance found in dark green and yellow fruits and vegetables (carrots, squash, green peppers, spinach) which the body converts into vitamin A. Carotene may inhibit the formation of cancer in the body.

Vitamin D helps control the absorption and use of calcium and phosphorous to build strong bones and teeth. It is found in fish-liver oils, fortified milk and margarine, and in small amounts in liver, egg yolks, and butter. It is called the "sunshine vitamin" because the skin can manufacture vitamin D if exposed to adequate sunlight. A deficiency of vitamin D causes adult rickets (osteomalacia).

Vitamin E is an antioxidant, which means that it

prevents the destruction of certain nutrients in the body and may retard cell aging. The best source of vitamin E is vegetable oils. It is also found in eggs, liver, green leafy vegetables, wheat germ, and nuts.

Vitamin K is necessary for normal blood clotting. It is found in liver, soybeans, and green leafy vegetables. The body manufactures about half of what it needs; the rest is obtained through diet.

WATER-SOLUBLE VITAMINS

Vitamin B complex (thiamine, riboflavin, niacin, pyridoxine, folic acid, B_{12}, biotin, pantothenic acid) is necessary for the activation of various enzymes in the cells and for a number of other cell functions including the metabolism of carbohydrates, protein, and fat.

1. *Thiamine* (B_1) is found in whole grain and enriched cereals and breads, pork, dry yeast, legumes, and green leafy vegetables. Thiamine deficiency causes beriberi, a disease of the nervous system, which is rare in the United States and is usually found here only in alcoholics.
2. *Riboflavin* (B_2) is found in milk, meat, cheese, eggs, whole grains, and green leafy vegetables, which are all good sources.
3. *Niacin* is found in whole grain and enriched breads and cereals, liver, lean meat, dry yeast, peanut butter, and legumes. Niacin deficiency causes pellagra, a skin disease which also in-

volves mental disorders and is rare in the United States.

4. *Pyridoxine* (B_6) is present in wheat germ, whole grains, liver and other red meats, peanuts, and soybeans.
5. *Folacin* (folic acid) is found in liver, green leafy vegetables, whole grains, legumes, orange juice, and nuts. Folic acid deficiency causes a type of anemia.
6. *Vitamin B_{12}* is found in liver, meat, eggs, milk, and cheese, which are the best sources. It is found only in animal products. Therefore, a vegetarian who eats *no* animal products may require a B_{12} supplement. Vitamin B_{12} deficiency may cause pernicious anemia.
7. *Biotin* is found in eggs, milk, meat, liver, legumes, yeast, chocolate, and nuts.
8. *Pantothenic acid* is present in egg yolks, liver, yeast, whole grains, potatoes, meat, salmon, broccoli, and peanuts.

Vitamin C contributes to tissue repair, wound healing, and the maintenance of blood vessels and capillaries by promoting the production of collagen, the most abundant protein in the body. It acts as a strong antioxidant, preventing the destruction of other nutrients both in the body and as a food additive. It also facilitates the absorption of iron and calcium in the body and may block the formation of cancer. Food sources of vitamin C include citrus fruits, stawberries, cantaloupe, tomatoes, green peppers, broccoli, cabbage, potatoes, and rose hips. Vitamin C is easily destroyed by heat. A deficiency of vitamin C causes scurvy.

Vitamin supplements are not necessary for people in reasonably good health who eat a variety of foods. These supplements provide only vitamins. On the other hand, food supplies protein, fat, carbohydrates, fiber, and minerals in addition to vitamins. Those who choose to eat a nutritionally deficient diet and take a vitamin supplement to make up for their poor eating habits are fooling themselves. Vitamins are only a small part of good nutrition and do not make up for poor or missed meals.

Vitamin supplements can be expensive, especially for those on a limited income. Taking excessive amounts of water-soluble vitamins is wasteful because the excess is excreted in the urine. Since fat-soluble vitamins are stored in the body, excessive amounts of them not only are wasteful but can cause serious health problems.

For example, high doses of vitamin A can cause jaundice and liver problems. Vitamin D is very toxic and can result in fractures, kidney damage, and hypertension. Excess vitamin K may interfere with blood clotting. Large doses of vitamin C may cause abdominal discomfort, gout, or kidney stones; block or increase the effect of medication; increase the ill effects of aspirin on the stomach; and give false results in the urine tests for sugar used by diabetics.

However, there are situations in which the requirements for vitamins are increased and in which a vitamin supplement may be appropriate. Surgery, an overactive thyroid, severe infection, burns, and stress increase the need for vitamin C and possibly for other vitamins. Intestinal illnesses and some medications may decrease vitamin absorption, and some chronic illnesses may require special diets or may limit the number of food choices available. Certain anemias require folate or vitamin B_{12} supplementation. In these cases, the appropriate supplement can be prescribed by the health care practitioner. Self-medication with vitamins is not advisable.

There have been reports of low-vitamin and other nutrient intake among older people whose diet consists of a limited number of foods (the tea-and-toast syndrome). In many cases, this type of deficiency can be corrected by eating a variety of foods, by paying attention to food choices, and especially by choosing nutritious foods over those composed of "empty" calories.

Heavy smoking, excessive alcohol intake, and severe stress increase the need for vitamin C. However, this need can usually be met by doubling the recommended dietary intake for vitamin C (drinking eight ounces of orange juice instead of four ounces, for example). There is no evidence that so-called stress vitamin supplements are of any value in coping with everyday stress. Eating a well-balanced diet is a better way to cope with stress.

Although much has been made of vitamin C's ability to fight the common cold, no reputable study has shown this to be true. So far, the best that can be said is that vitamin C *may* lessen the severity of cold symptoms in some people.

Self-medication with vitamins can be both wasteful and hazardous. In addition, many over-the-counter vitamin supplements contain haphazard amounts of different vitamins. (There may be one-half the daily requirement for one vitamin and five times the daily requirement for another.) "Megadoses" (ten times the Recommended Dietary Allowance) of vitamins may be helpful in some very rare diseases, but because they can be very dangerous they should *never* be used without the advice and knowledge of your health care practitioner.

Some foods are fortified or enriched with certain nutrients. Originally this was done to overcome some populationwide deficiency which was a public health problem; for example, the addition of iodine to table salt to prevent goiter. Now many manufacturers voluntarily add vitamins and other nutrients to food products which ordinarily would not be considered appropriate food choices, like processed food or candy bars, in order to make "empty" calories seem nutritious. Others add vitamins to items such as highly sugared cereals to increase their desirability. This is false nutrition, since these foods are still high in fat, sugar, and calories as well as being expensive. This practice is also profitable for the manufacturer, since adding a penny's worth of vitamins easily raises the price charged for the item by twenty or thirty cents. A well-balanced diet is still the best source of nutrients.

To preserve vitamins in foods:

1. Eat fresh foods as soon as possible after purchasing them.
2. Store ripe fruit and vegetables in the refrigerator; store potatoes, cereals, and rice in a cool, dark place.
3. Keep milk in an opaque container (riboflavin is destroyed by light).
4. Wash vegetables and fruits quickly just before eating them. Eat them raw, steamed, or cooked rapidly in a very small amount of water.
5. Eat potatoes with their skins.
6. Do not cook vegetables with baking soda—it destroys thiamine and vitamin C.

A great deal of research is in progress exploring new uses for vitamins in areas such as the prevention and treatment of cancer, arthritis, and other illnesses. However, claims made on the basis of preliminary data are not valid, since they may be disproved by additional research. While it is important to keep abreast of the latest developments, it is not wise to attempt to bring about radical or miracle cures with vitamins or any medication or treatment unless there is very good evidence that you are not wasting your time and money on something which is worthless or could even be harmful.

MINERALS:
Approximately twenty-two minerals are neces-

sary for good health; they contribute to a variety of body functions in the cells, bones, nerves, and the enzyme systems. Among these minerals are calcium, phosphorous, sodium, iron, zinc, copper, and selenium. Several minerals have already been discussed earlier in this chapter; however, two topics are worth mentioning here.

Iron. This mineral is a necessary component of hemoglobin, the portion of the red blood cell which carries oxygen. Many older people have low dietary iron intakes because of poor food choices and/or a limited income. Iron deficiency anemia is the most common form of anemia among older people.

Iron is not well absorbed by the body. Foods high in calcium and vitamin C increase absorption; foods high in phosphorous, oxalic and phytic acids (found in spinach and legumes), and the food additive EDTA reduce its absorption. The best food sources for iron are meat, liver, and whole grains. Iron is also found in eggs, fortified breads and cereals, legumes, raisins, and green leafy vegetables. Taking iron supplements without the knowledge and advice of your health care practitioner can be harmful, since toxic amounts can be stored in the body, damaging the liver and the heart.

Trace minerals. Most of the minerals required by the body, such as zinc, copper, and selenium, are called microminerals or trace minerals because only very small amounts of them are necessary to maintain health. There is often a very small difference between the safe level required for good health and a toxic amount. Therefore, mineral supplements

83

can be quite dangerous and should not be taken without professional advice.

Health Problems Related to Nutrition

CONSTIPATION:

Constipation plagues many older people. Some people think that they must have a bowel movement every day to keep healthy. However, many normal, healthy people have a bowel movement only once every two or three days; others may have more than one a day. Constipation occurs not only when bowel movements are too infrequent but also when stools are hard, dry, and difficult to pass.

Constipation has many causes, including the decreased intestinal muscle tone associated with aging, abuse of laxatives, a low-fiber diet, low fluid intake, inactivity and lack of exercise, an illness such as diabetes or a sluggish thyroid gland, depression, and certain medications. With painful hemorrhoids or other rectal problems, the urge to have a bowel movement may be ignored. Older people, especially those with chronic health problems, use a lot of medications, and many of these contribute to constipation. Some examples are antacids which contain aluminum; codeine, some tranquilizers, sedatives, diuretics ("water pills"), and antidiarrhea preparations.

If you are troubled with chronic constipation, visit your health care practitioner for a checkup. A previously undiagnosed illness or long-term medication use for another health problem may be the cause.

To prevent constipation you can do a number of things:

1. Drink at least six glasses of liquid a day, preferably water. Prune juice may also be helpful. If you take bran, adequate fluid intake is especially important to prevent a stool impaction.
2. Increase the amount of fiber (roughage) in your diet by eating plenty of raw fruits, vegetables, and whole grain products.
3. Establish a regular time for a bowel movement; many people find after breakfast to be most convenient.
4. Get some type of exercise daily. The sedentary life promotes constipation. Walking is an appropriate form of exercise and usually fits easily into a daily routine.
5. Do not depend on laxatives. Their constant use may decrease nutrient and medication absorption in the intestines while also decreasing their normal muscle tone and responsiveness. Over-the-counter laxatives may contain harsh or irritating ingredients. If an occasional laxative is necessary, it should be prescribed by your health care practitioner.

CANCER AND DIET:

For years there has been much discussion about various foods being linked to different types of cancer or, conversely, offering protection from cancer. Some of these links appear to be worth further consideration; others are questionable.

Two government agencies, the National Cancer Institute (1979) and the National Academy of Sciences (1982), in reviewing current research about the relationship between cancer and diet, have issued general recommendations for dietary changes which may help lower the risk of cancer. These are:

1. Decrease the amount of dietary fats consumed (both saturated and unsaturated fats). The high-fat diet appears to be associated with cancer of both the breast and the colon.
2. Decrease consumption of salt-cured, pickled, and smoked foods.
3. Increase consumption of fruits and vegetables, especially those which contain vitamin C and vitamin A. Studies have indicated that both these vitamins may prevent cancer formation. Vitamin C foods include citrus fruits, strawberries, tomatoes, papaya, green peppers, broccoli, and potatoes. Vitamin A sources include green leafy or orange vegetables. Vegetables of the mustard family—broccoli, brussels sprouts, cabbage, cauliflower, kale— were particularly singled out as being related to a decreased rate of stomach, colon, and rectal cancer.
4. Increase consumption of whole grain breads and cereals. Dietary fiber (also found in fresh

fruits and vegetables) may decrease the risk of colon cancer.

5. Limit alcohol intake to one or two drinks a day. Heavy alcohol consumption is associated with cancer of the mouth, throat, esophagus, larynx, and liver, especially in smokers.
6. Maintain ideal weight. Obesity is associated with cancer of the breast and of the lining of the uterus.

Evidence of cancer caused by food additives such as nitrates and saccharin, while suggestive, is not conclusive. However, it seems prudent to keep intake of these substances to a minimum.

There may also be a relationship between high-protein intake and cancer, but neither agency has made any specific recommendations as of this time. However, scientists have noted that the average American diet is two to three times higher in protein than is recommended. (Protein should make up approximately 12 percent of caloric intake.)

Safety

Accidents are a major cause of death in the United States, yet they are largely preventable. This statistic, of course, includes the appalling number of automobile-related deaths which are not primarily the concern of older people, although we, too, contribute our share of these fatalities.

Falls are the chief late-life accident menace, with burns, electric shock, and other traumas following.

Most of these accidents occur at home, and although generally not immediately fatal, they can lead to fatal complications. Following are the most common menaces, indoors and out, and ways to circumvent them.

THE DARK:

As we grow older, our vision may grow less acute, and we tend to be awake more often during the dark hours. To prevent accidents, survey your surroundings to find unlit areas which you use frequently, particularly where there are steps or carpet edges, and light them. If you leave your bed during the night, have a bed light at hand and turn it on. Use a low-watt baseboard plug-in light close to your bed if a bed light wakes your spouse.

SCATTER RUGS:

These should be either retired or firmly affixed to the floor with their edges taped down.

STEPS AND STAIRS:

In addition to adequate lighting, steps and stairs should have hand rails, and the hand rails should be used. Bifocal glasses make negotiating stairs particularly difficult, so that special care should be taken.

FLOORS:

Use nonslip floor waxes; avoid soft-soled slippers; and wear well-fitted shoes with nonskid or rubber soles.

MOVABLE OBJECTS:

Chairs, stools, occasional tables, and electric cords are sometimes moved for special occasions and not returned to their accustomed places. Such moves can cause falls or bruises. Pets can also get in the way; be aware of them. Keep your surroundings as stable as possible to prevent accidents.

BATHTUBS:

These are slippery when wet and should have hand rails and nonslip strips or mats. Getting out of the tub can be a difficult feat for some older people and should be undertaken carefully. Shower stalls are safer and easier to negotiate. Bathtub stools are available and often helpful.

LADDERS AND STEPSTOOLS:

If you need to climb, use strong, well-built ladders and stepstools which are firmly anchored to the floor, not other furnishings such as chairs, tables, windowsills, or shelves which happen to be nearby. Try not to climb at all when you are alone in a house. Store often used objects within normal reach.

ICE:

A six-inch patch of ice can be just as lethal as a smoothly frozen lake if you happen to hit it wrong. When there is ice or snow on the ground, take extreme care when venturing outside, even to the back steps. It is better to wait, if possible, until nature or public maintenance has removed the threat. Falling on ice can be deadly to young and old alike.

CURBS, RUTS, POTHOLES, AND OTHER OUTDOOR HAZARDS:

While walking out-of-doors, look where you are stepping, even though looking at trees, hilltops, or the sky may be more pleasurable.

Most important, older people should try not to hurry as they go about daily rounds. Allow enough time to do what you have to do without unaccustomed haste. Don't run for trains or buses. The time you save may wind you up in a hospital intensive-care unit.

If a cane ("sticks," as inveterate users call them) can be helpful, use it.

BURNS AND SHOCKS:

Living without electricity is almost unimaginable to most twentieth-century Western people, but electricity, carelessly used, can cause serious accidents through shock or fire, largely at home.

House wiring should be checked regularly, and cords leading to appliances kept in good condition. Portable lamp cords should be kept away from frequented areas. Heating pads should be on "low" during sleep, and heating units should not be at floor level.

Smoking in bed is inviting a painful death!

POISONOUS OR TOXIC SUBSTANCES:

If your eyesight is not the best, all poisonous or

toxic substances should be clearly marked and kept in specific areas so that they will not be ingested in error.

Potentially dangerous chemicals are commonly used in our daily living—insect sprays, paint removers, cleaning fluids, and so forth. Warning labels should be carefully read and followed.

DRIVING:

Three physical disabilities militate against older persons continuing to drive: defective vision, defective hearing, and severe hypertension. Follow your health care practitioner's advice when it's time to renew your driver's license. Aging tends to slow reactions slightly, but in good drivers this shortcoming is fully compensated for by experience. "Older, fit drivers are the least dangerous on the road," Alex Comfort asserts in *A Good Age*.

Fasten your seat belt when you get behind the wheel. Most serious accidents occur within twenty miles of home.

TEMPERATURE:

As our bodies age they become less efficient at adjusting to hot or cold weather. Our responses to heat and cold may also be affected by such illnesses as heart disease or diabetes, or by medications such as tranquilizers.

In hot weather avoid strenuous exercise and wear light, loose-fitting clothing which allows perspiration to evaporate. Drink plenty of fluids, especially water and juices. Salt tablets are not recommended unless specifically prescribed by a health care practitioner. If nausea, dizziness, weakness, or headache occur, they may be the first symptoms of heat exhaustion or heat stroke and should not be ignored.

Older people, especially those who are chronically ill, who have faulty body temperature regulating mechanisms, or who do not try to stay warm in cold weather, risk developing accidental hypothermia. This is a condition in which the body temperature (usually around 98° F) falls to 95° F or below. Symptoms of accidental hypothermia include confusion, sluggishness, and very slow respiration and heartbeat. If the body temperature regulating system is not working properly, the affected person may not even shiver or feel cold. Accidental hypothermia may be fatal if it is not recognized. Treatment must begin immediately and consists of gradual rewarming of the body under close medical supervision, usually in a hospital.

However, prevention is the first line of defense. Therefore, in cold weather it is a good idea to keep the thermostat at no lower than 65° F. Dress warmly, both indoors and out, and remember that several thin layers of clothing are warmer than one thick layer. At night use enough blankets, or an electric blanket at "low" setting, to keep warm in bed. Eat regular meals and remain as active as possible. If housebound, keep in touch with a family member, a neighbor, or a friend daily by telephone.

Sleep

The amount of sleep we need changes throughout our lifetimes. Infants and children need much more sleep than do adults, and older adults apparently require less sleep than do younger adults. Sleep also seems to be lighter, with more frequent awakenings when we are older. However, the number of hours slept is not as important as whether one feels rested the next day. Five or six hours of sleep may be enough for some, while others may need eight hours.

Everyone has experienced occasional difficulty in falling asleep. This is often caused by anxiety over one of life's problems—financial woes, a job interview, a sick child—and sleep returns to normal after the crisis has passed. Some people, however, are troubled by chronic insomnia for weeks, months, or even years.

Sleep disturbances have a variety of causes. One of the most important is a sedentary life style which, unfortunately, is all too common today. Inactivity leads to boredom and apathy, not to a good night's sleep! Regular exercise, on the other hand, is invigorating, promotes relaxation, and improves sleep.

Afternoon naps are another culprit. It is difficult to sleep six or eight hours at night when one naps for two or three hours during the day. Often, the elimination of the afternoon nap will promote a restful night's sleep. If you insist on taking an afternoon nap, remember that you may not sleep as long or as well at night.

Caffeine is a stimulant. It wakes you up and makes you feel more alert—not the effect that you want if you are trying to fall asleep. Therefore, avoid caffeine-containing beverages such as coffee, tea, or cola drinks in the evening or at bedtime. If you drink several cups of coffee or tea a day, cut down on your consumption. Some people find that they cannot tolerate any caffeine drinks and that they sleep much better if they eliminate them.

Other causes of sleeping problems are certain illnesses (e.g., an overactive thyroid, breathing difficulties), medications (some cardiac or thyroid drugs), environmental factors (noise, a hot room), overuse or abuse of sleeping medications, and depression associated with early morning awakening.

SLEEP MEDICATIONS:

Some women rely on medications to help them sleep. The most commonly used medications include barbiturates, tranquilizers, and over-the-counter drugs.

Such barbiturate drugs as secobarbitol (Seconal) are dangerous medications because they can be addictive and cause unpleasant withdrawal symptoms if stopped abruptly. Milder sleep medications like flurazepam (Dalmane) are more commonly used today. However, even with the use of milder medications, emotional and physical dependence can develop. Long-term use of sleep medications is counterproductive, since in many people they disturb normal sleeping patterns and increase the insomnia they were supposed to correct. They can also cause daytime drowsiness, confusion, and decrease in alertness. Accidental or intentional overdose, especially when combined with alcohol, can lead to death.

Over-the-counter sleeping aids are also not to be taken lightly. Some may cause dry mouth or blurred vision. They may interact or interfere with medications, taken for other illnesses, causing unpleasant side effects. They may also adversely affect such illnesses as high blood pressure.

That said, it is true that some medications may be useful in relieving insomnia. For example, if depression is found to be the cause, appropriate treatment may include antidepressant medication. Other illnesses such as an overactive thyroid, when treated with the appropriate medication, may relieve insomnia. However, sleeping medications should be used only by those who really need them and then only for a short time (two to four weeks) and only under the careful guidance of a health care practitioner.

SUGGESTIONS FOR A GOOD NIGHT'S SLEEP:
1. Establish a regular pattern. Go to sleep at approximately the same time each night and get up at about the same time each morning.
2. Eliminate afternoon naps.
3. Avoid caffeine drinks (coffee, tea, colas), especially in the evening. Instead, have that time-honored bedtime drink, a glass of warm milk. It is a relaxing alternative.

4. Have a light, nourishing evening meal instead of a big dinner. Avoid rich or fatty foods.
5. Exercise, outdoors if possible, every day.
6. Relax in the evening with a warm bath, meditation, some pleasant reading. Make a quiet time for yourself.
7. Make your surroundings as comfortable as possible. Bedrooms should not be too warm and should be well ventilated and protected from outside noise if possible.

Stress

Stress may be defined as anything which affects the body's normal equilibrium or steady state. Excitement, fear, tension, or pleasure affect this steady state by causing such responses as rapid heartbeat, sweaty palms, and increased alertness.

We usually think of stress in negative terms, but stress is not necessarily negative. For example, many types of exercise stress the body and in doing so strengthen the heart and lungs and improve muscle tone and circulation. Athletes find that getting "up" for a game improves their concentration and performance. We become excited in anticipation of a long-awaited vacation or a visit from loved ones. These are different types of what can be called positive stress.

We could not survive without any stresses in our lives. Some stress is necessary for normal physical and emotional health. Negative stresses such as worry, fear, anxiety, and frustration are also a normal part of living. However, chronic stress—an excessive amount of negative stress over long periods of time—can cause serious problems.

Normal responses to negative physical or emotional stress include "upset stomach," stiff neck, headache, fatigue, and mild depression (feeling "blue"). Usually these responses are temporary and disappear when the problem causing the stress is relieved. However, constant and excessive stresses can cause these bodily responses to continue and may thus contribute to physical and emotional illness. Medical evidence implies that even continued stress by itself does not cause illness but that, in combination with other factors such as heredity, environment, nutrition, exercise, and other health habits, it may predispose one to a particular illness.

It is easy to see the link with stress in illness which are often made worse by emotional upset such as asthma, severe depression, colitis, and migraine headache. Chronic stress may also play a role in serious illnesses such as heart disease, high blood pressure, peptic ulcer, and cancer. This is an area of active research; much is still to be learned. However, it is certainly wise to take steps to reduce and control continued negative stresses in life.

STRESS OVERLOAD:

Constant or excessive stresses may lead to stress overload. We may feel overwhelmed by situations that we have handled easily in the past, or we may respond much more intensely to a minor incident or problem than we usually would. Our ability to complete tasks and to deal effectively with problems may decrease. If this kind of tension and anxiety is not relieved, we may respond with an exacerbation of our "normal" stress response—such as severe depression, frequent migraine headaches, or constant diarrhea. Obviously, treating these types of illness involves treating or alleviating the basic cause of the stress.

HOW TO COPE WITH STRESS:
1. *Listen to your body.* Learn to recognize the first signs of stress in your body so that you can deal with stress more effectively.
2. *Learn to say no.* Too often we think that we must be all things to all people, that we must take charge of everything and do it all ourselves. Let others share responsibility and do not commit yourself if you do not have the time or energy.
3. *Do not place unrealistic expectations on yourself.* This leads only to frustration.
4. *Take time for recreation.* Sports, hobbies, the theater, movies, and books all provide a break from the everyday grind.
5. *Get enough sleep.* A person who is well rested is better able to cope.
6. *Work off tension with physical exercise.* Regular exercise is a good outlet for stress in addition to keeping one fit.
7. *Be flexible.*
8. *Talk the problem over with someone.* None of us can handle all our problems by ourselves

all the time. An emphathetic friend, relative, or health professional can provide a sounding board as well as needed support and guidance.

9. *Be prudent about medication.* Tranquilizers and sedatives administered by a qualified health practitioner can be useful in combating the effects of severe stress when used on a short-term basis. However, medication should not be used as a crutch to avoid dealing with the problem causing the stress. Never take medication prescribed for someone else.

10. *Take a vacation occasionally.* A complete change of scenery helps put things in perspective as well as providing relaxation.

11. *Take time for yourself.* A quiet time alone, even if only for a few minutes, can help you relax. Some people find yoga, meditation and deep breathing helpful in promoting relaxation.

TIMETABLE FOR PHYSICAL EXAMINATION AND IMMUNIZATION
Women Age 55 and Over

Examination	Suggested Frequency
General physical examination	Every 5 years until age 59
	Every 2 years after age 60
Blood pressure check	Once a year
Eye examination including glaucoma testing	Once a year
Breast self-examination	Once a month
Breast examination (by health care practitioner)	Once a year
Pelvic examination	Once a year
Pap smear	Once every 1 to 3 years*
Dental examination	Once or twice a year
Mammography	Once a year after age 50

*Pap smears are recommended once every three years after two negative yearly tests by the American Cancer Society. This recommendation is considered controversial by some experts.

Note: This suggested schedule is for healthy women without symptoms and at normal risk. If you have a chronic illness or are at a high risk for an illness, you may require more frequent examinations. If you have symptoms of illness, you should consult a health care practitioner as soon as possible.

Rectal examination	Once a year
Test for blood in stool	Once a year
Proctosigmoidoscopy	Every 3 to 5 years after age 50, after 2 negative yearly tests
Endometrial tissue sample	At menopause for women on estrogen therapy or with a history of infertility, failure to ovulate, abnormal uterine bleeding

Immunization	**Suggested Frequency**
Influenza (flu) vaccine	Once a year over age 65
	Once a year for anyone with a chronic illness such as heart disease, pulmonary disease, diabetes
Pneumonia vaccine	Once every 3 to 4 years over age 65 or for those with a chronic illness
Diphtheria and tetanus vaccine	Once every 10 years
Smallpox vaccine	Not necessary unless traveling to certain high-risk areas

THREE

Mental Health
Goals for
Older Women

EMOTIONAL CHALLENGES IN FACING CHANGE AND LOSS

In an essay on being old, "The Measure of My Days," Florida Scott-Maxwell writes:

> We who are old know that age is more than a disability. It is an intense and varied experience, almost beyond our capacity at times, but something to be carried on high. If it is a loud defeat, it is also a victory, meaningful for the initiates of time, if not for those who have come less far.

Today, because we older women live in a society that dismisses our strengths and dwells on our weaknesses, turning "defeat" into "victory" is an uphill battle but one that can be won. Growing old is not for sissies.

The timid among us resist change, but change is the name of the game as we grow older—change that more often than not translates into loss—personal, physical, and economic. How can we cope with these changes? First of all by facing them and then, with the help of our accumulated experience and wisdom, continuing to grow with them.

On Our Own

English people sometimes say that we are "on our own" rather than "alone"—a phrase that expresses a sense of freedom and independence instead of loneliness and isolation. As we grow older, we find ourselves more and more "on our own." People close to us move away, become ill, or die—friends, relatives, parents, and, most painfully, spouses. Although the death of anyone close to us, particularly if he or she has lived with or near us, can be devastating, the death of a spouse is said to cause the greatest stress in the human condition.

Some caregivers speak of "grief work" as a timetable for grieving, of specified periods for "numbness," "anger," "depression," and "acceptance," implying that the bereaved should at some particular time "recover" and be ready to begin a "new life." We believe that bereaved people don't recover from grief but rather adjust to it and are then ready for that new life. The time this takes and the way it is done depends on the individual.

American novelist Shirley Hazzard's heroine in *The Bay of Noon* speaks of her loss:

When people say of their tragedies, "I don't often think of it now," what they mean is it has entered permanently into their thoughts, and colors everything. Because the idea of [Gaetano] is always with me, I'm less shocked now, when I suddenly come upon some reminder of him, than I was long ago when he still seemed *a grief I must get over.*

There is grief work to be done, but since every bereaved person is different there can be no standard prescription for adjustment. Unfortunately, our culture denies the bereaved the "trappings of woe" and, after a brief period, expects us to act and even feel as we always have. The timetable theory indicates that if we grieve too long we are in "trouble," perhaps even mentally ill. If we believe this, we may become frightened and depressed.

Many of us need to grieve for months or even years. After all, the loss of someone who has been uppermost in one's thoughts for the large part of a lifetime cannot be accepted and adjusted to in a trice. Sometimes we find former relationships with friends and children whom we love difficult because they cannot share our pain. Those who have been there and who have adjusted to some degree can often help us more than anyone else. In response to this need, successful self-help programs for widows have evolved throughout the country.

Grief work can also mean facing negative feelings of anger, frustration, and guilt which must be let out of the dark closets of our minds, examined, accepted, and placed in perspective. We often need professional help to do this.

While grieving is acute, whether we express it or not, we are becoming a "new person" on our own, and we must face day-to-day living. If we have been dependent on others, doing this alone can be staggeringly difficult. If we have always been independent, these details may trouble us less and even distract us from the emptiness inside. In either case, help is available through widow and other counseling programs. The more independent among us may, in time, wish to help others.

The problems facing the older widow are different from those of younger women who, like Lynne Caine, author of the sensitive and self-revealing book *Widow,* slowly and painfully work toward a new beginning. Older widows seldom remarry and often find it difficult or impossible to live with children, relatives, or friends. They are, therefore, faced with learning to live alone, as are many divorced women, whose problems are discussed in detail in Chapter 5.

Many older widows in the 1980s had never spent a night alone until their husbands were hospitalized or died. In the traditional way of the first half of this century, these women lived with their parents until they married, and neither they nor their husbands were away from home alone, even overnight. Now being alone may be their lot, and most say that loneliness is their greatest problem. How does one live with this aching loneliness, which Patricia O'Brien in her book, *A Woman Alone,* defines as "carnivorous self-absorption," and learn appreciation of solitude, an ability to accept and live with oneself without fear? The actress Helen Hayes, now in her eighties, after fifteen years of widowhood, said, "Solitude—walking alone, doing things alone—is the most blessed thing in the world. And

I think I am beginning to find myself a little bit."

In a perceptive chapter, "Living," O'Brien distinguishes between women who react to aloneness by building and those who merely cope. The builders are usually blessed with a positive self-image and face enforced aloneness as a challenge from which good may be wrung. The copers, she implies, merely survive.

She goes on to say that women on their own who build are usually planners. One widow, whose husband's long terminal illness forced her to plan for a life on her own and whose income from her own efforts shields her from the poverty that is the lot of so many older widows, planned to do the things that her husband didn't like—live in the city, entertain, listen to classical music, go to way-out films, and travel to far-off, uncomfortable places. While her program has not brought the relief from pain that she had hoped, she lives a good life. Too, she has actively, though not always successfully, sought the blessings of solitude extolled by Miss Hayes. This woman is a planner, and though her friends laugh at her "little black book" in which she writes down all these doings, it is her constant companion and security blanket.

For women alone, O'Brien continues,

There is no structure that will generate things happening if they don't make them happen, unlike the household of a woman with children (now fondly and rosily remembered by many older widows) where the daily routine means a variety of expected and unexpected events . . . a mixture of warmth and worry.

However, this very freedom to plan and build must be controlled lest it become self-destructive license.

On the other hand, "sufficient unto the day is the evil thereof." While widows may plan events ahead to keep their lives in motion, they must also learn to take each day, good and bad, as it comes and know that it too will pass.

The closing lines of Linda Paston's moving yet humorous poem, "The Five Stages of Grief," expresses it all:

> Acceptance. I finally reach it.
> But something is wrong.
> Grief is a circular staircase.
> I have lost you.

These are some practical guidelines which may help newly widowed older women accept grief and loneliness and adjust to them.

1. Remember as much and weep as much, and as often as you feel the need until the pain eases. If your family and friends seem to tire of it and you, seek the help and company of other widows who have been there. You are not alone.
2. Don't follow well-meaning advice and make irrevocable decisions too soon. Wait until you have adjusted enough to think clearly.

3. If you need to, seek help from qualified persons for the dailiness of living—driving, shopping, banking, budgeting, etc.—and for your emotional pain.
4. Reexamine your social relationships only when you have adjusted to your grief and your status as a person alone. Very often new relationships prove more satisfying than old ones because you are a new person "on your own."
5. When you sense joy, satisfaction, and hope—be glad, not guilty—for this is what the person who loved you would want for you.

Unhappily, the loss of your spouse or the person to whom you have been closest is not always the final bereavement for older people. We live on a shrinking planet. In *You and Your Aging Parent*, Barbara Silverstone speaks of the dismay of an adult child at her father's wildly grieving reaction to the death of a pet bird shortly after his wife's death. It was not that he mourned for the little pet *too much* but that now there was *too much loss* to be borne! As we grow older, so do our contemporaries, old friends and new alike, and they move away, become physically ill or just impossible, and they die. So, sometimes, do grown children, the "unkindest cut of all," for this loss is against nature. Indeed, growing old is not for sissies!

Time on Our Hands

In our puritan work-ethic society, the word "leisure" has a negative connotation. It should not be so. A contributor to a perceptive collection of essays, *Time on Our Hands*, writes, "To be at leisure is not to be on vacation from reality. Leisure is the time for discovery . . . the occasion for learning and freedom, for rest and restoration." In the same work, another writer maintains that "leisure is becoming a major human enterprise in a technological culture," and "the retired person is the pivotal agent for change. Far from having no significance s(he) is the pioneer prophet of tomorrow."

Whether a woman continues her full-time job as a housewife into "olderhood" or has gone to work at some point in her life, the demands on her time lessen as she grows older. This diminution may be seen as another loss to cope with or as a challenge to become that "pioneer prophet of tomorrow."

Despite myths to the contrary, many women do become very committed to their paid jobs, and retirement can be a shock. Many of these retirees now widowed are not returning to their former occupations as full-time housewives and caregivers but, rather, facing living alone with more time on their hands and much less money in their pockets. But if retire we must, there are compensations:

We no longer have to march to another's drum.
Our time is our own, to cultivate and make
    flower as we will.
We can spend more time with the people we
    love and not necessarily those we serve.
We can pursue those way-out interests that

intrigued us along the way—watercoloring,
orchid culture, yoga, reading lots of books.
It's our own ball game.

We can spend more time and energy cultivating
ourselves—our often neglected minds and
bodies.

Once in awhile, we can even stay in bed longer
on a cold winter morning!

In addition to the opportunities for personal growth open to us through fulfilling pleasure or continued learning, there is a whole world that needs us as trained and expert volunteers and committed advocates for social and political change. The choices are limitless.

Diminishing Returns

There can be no question, in view of the previously discussed inequalities in government and private pension provisions for women and the seemingly irreversible inflation with which we are faced, that most older retired and/or widowed women have less money than they used to have.

These "diminishing returns" are relative. Women who have always been poor may now be nearly destitute and thus become society's responsibility. The quality of their future life will depend upon their own willingness and ability to accept without false pride the help which is owed them.

Those who were well off in mid-life may have to learn to do with a lot less. Being widowed and on our own may mean learning for the first time to plan and operate our dwindling financial affairs and to hone our slimming budgets. It should also mean long-range and not especially pleasant planning for a future in which we may no longer be able to care for ourselves.

Fortunately, most women have taken some part in managing family finances, if only to make do on a weekly household allowance. Unfortunately, many know little or nothing about such perplexing matters as personal banking, investments (with their endless and complex options), credit, mortgages, rentals, taxes, pensions, wills, and the like. Some of us have relatives and/or friends qualified and willing to advise and support us with regard to at least some of these problems. Public and private resources are also available.

Womanpower

"Power" was a man's word, but we women have possessed it, used and misused it, and feel that we lose it as we grow older. Some of the most powerful political rulers in the history of the West have been women—Hatshepsut, Cleopatra, Elizabeth I, Catherine the Great, Maria Theresa, Queen Victoria. Victoria, possibly the most powerful individual of her time (1837–1901), through her personal way of living and moral code increased the powerlessness of women of the late nineteenth and early twentieth centuries. The "feminine mystique" which imprisoned them in their homes or sweatshops was labeled and decried by Betty Friedan in the 1960s and has been largely demythologized by today's women's movement.

Power to most of us older women in the 1980s has been channeled through the men in our lives—husbands, colleagues, friends. Although we may have been unaware that we were wielding power, when it dwindles through our fading abilities to attract and influence and our men disappear, we sense its loss and feel diminished by it. As we are getting to know ourselves better, however, we begin to suspect that this manipulation of men was not power at all but a cop-out, born of not knowing, and that we must look inside ourselves for the real source of power. We know that we must keep control of our own lives as long as we can and enjoy the lessening of responsibility for others' lives that growing older can bring.

If we are losing power and even control as individuals, we are gaining it as a group. As the number of us older women increases and our educational level and political knowhow rises, our potential clout is becoming formidable. How we can use this collective power for our own good is the subject of the section on advocacy later on in this chapter.

More frightening to us older women on our own than loss of power or control over our own or other's lives is a sense of our expendability, of not being needed at all. O'Brien feels that this fear is a "Source of a deep and desolating loneliness in some women . . . an engulfing vacuum that comes from a loss of interconnection with other people." Becoming "expendable" is believed by some to be the basic human fear. This emptiness, which troubles most people at times, can be filled by constantly remembering that we are not really alone and that we are responsible to those who love us, to our community, and most importantly to ourselves.

Old Can Be Beautiful

Nowhere is sexism more rampant than in the contrasting ways older men and older women are seen by others and consequently by themselves. Because the physical attributes of youth are equated with beauty in the female, the older woman is dismissed, whereas an older man may be said to be "interesting," "distinguished," and even "handsome."

An older woman we admire says that nothing turns her off so much as being told, "You must have been beautiful when you were young." "I am still beautiful," she says, "if I ever was, but in a different way." And she is insulted when given the old saw, "You haven't changed a bit." "Not changed," she exclaims, "by all the learning and living I have done!"

Until we are forty or so, it has been said that our "looks" are given to us and that afterward their future, good or bad, is up to us. This responsibility means not only good skin care, exercise, and nutrition, important as these are, but how we think and feel inside ourselves. Laugh lines are more attractive than furrowed brows, and a straight, proud carriage is more attractive than a discouraged slump.

We older women must redefine beauty as an inner grace that is reflected in our outer appearance and continue to walk proud.

Aging Is Not a Disease

Only in the last twenty years, as our aging population has grown so dramatically, have *geriatrics* (a branch of medicine dealing with the specific diseases of old age) and *gerontology* (the study of the process of aging) concerned the medical and allied health professions. As a result of studies and deliberations, the medical profession has concluded that aging is not in itself a disease but rather that diseases behave differently and must be treated differently in aging people and that certain diseases are more common among them than among younger people. As children are not physiologically just small adults, so aging people are not physiologically just older adults.

To help us handle some of these diseases, should they occur, the following chapter discusses the older woman *vis-à-vis* today's health care system and the problems most often occurring among us.

And at the End

We all must die, some at an earlier age than others. We who have survived into olderhood know that the end cannot be too far off, but, because most of us have looked on the face of death and thought a great deal about it, we may dread it less than we did when we were younger.

It is the manner of our going that worries us. We hope that it will be quick, painless, and without fear. But, for some of us, this will not be; we ask that, as a dying person, we be treated with honesty, compassion, and respect.

COPING AND BUILDING

To Know and Respect Ourselves

A friend who is aware of our interest in "successful aging" writes:

> In a month my graduating class at Smith will celebrate its fiftieth reunion. I will not be there, but on a bright weekend at the first of May, I spent an hour on the campus by myself.
>
> I walked past unchanged classroom buildings and a much larger library, past the assembly hall where we attended required, non-sectarian chapel, to my freshman dormitory. Then I walked down the steep path to the edge of lovely, unchanged Paradise Pond. Four girls and a boy had come galloping down behind me to play on the swings along the path. I could hear their young, high voices, their giggles and the sound of a musical instrument they had brought with them. In the background, a tom-tom beat at some spring festival further away.
>
> I sat on the grass and looked at the water and trees.

For a strange moment, I became a girl again, wanting to get on with my life, not quite sure how.

After a while, I looked at my watch. My hour had gone. When I stood up, I was stiff but I knew the young, restless, energetic person I had been had grown well, had become full of treasures massed through the day-in, day-out business of living.

The people I have known have added to my life and become part of it—lovers, children, friends, colleagues, even enemies; the places I have visited and loved, as near as Amherst, Massachusetts, as far away as China; the work I have done; all I have learned, am still learning; the little things that have made me laugh or cry or lose my temper; and the joys and sorrows too deep for laughter, tears, or anger. I want to know more, do more, see more; but I am content. I am proud of the way I have used my life. I like being seventy. My accumulated years become me well.

These are the words of a strong and fortunate woman who has put her past and her future together and reached what the psychologist Erik Erikson called "integrity," the final task in human development.

Paul Douglas wrote in *The Fullness of Time*, "The old have more going for them than is normally assumed. New growth, new directions lie open for those willing to suffer the growing pains of a second adolescence."

According to Robert Butler, one of today's leading professional spokesmen for older people, "A major developmental task in old age is to *clarify, deepen,* and *find use for* what one has already attained in a lifetime of learning and adapting." He continues by listing the ways in which he believes older people go about this task: through a changed sense of time with a sensory enjoyment of the here and now; through a sense of continuity in the life cycle; through a "life review" in which past conflicts may be resolved in one's mind and past joys remembered; through a cherishing of familiar objects; through an ability to pass to others that which is worthy in one's life; through knowing when to forego power; and finally through a capacity for continuing growth.

At any age, since no two persons are alike nor their circumstances the same, these developmental stages and tasks can serve only as guideposts. The way we go depends upon us, since each of us must find our own answers, but the qualities we must bring with us to our older years seem to be courage, self-knowledge, self-respect, and the ability to grow.

Margaret Huyck writes, "Life will always be full of strife, anxiety and challenge. These can be experienced as paralyzing or as creating opportunities for growth."

To Change Motivations and Patterns of Living

Throughout our lives, we have marched to another's drum—that of parents, teachers, husbands, children, bosses; and we have answered to social imperatives—success in school, in our homes, in our jobs—to the approval and approbation of our peers. Now we are free!

We get out of bed in the morning because we want to—because the sun is shining, it's spring, summer, winter, fall; or we are hungry; or the plants need watering; or we want the answer to yesterday's crossword puzzle in today's papers; or our backs ache less when we are standing up. The reasons are many but they are all for us.

Once up and about, living can be very full for us older women on our own. As we became busier in earlier years, we may never have had time for the things that moved us or that we dreamed of when we were very young. There are so many books not read or not written, music not heard or not played, sights not seen, friendships not tended.

When we are older, although we may have more time, some of us have less energy. So perhaps we should take longer to do the jobs we have set for ourselves, move more slowly, enjoy what we are doing at the moment rather than rushing on to what we are going to do next. Rushing seems to be a way of our American culture. In many older societies people move at a more leisurely pace.

We should set some flexible rules for our living. First and most important, we must keep our physical wellness to the best of our abilities, following, perhaps, the guidelines in Chapter 2, "Maintaining Wellness." We should not set unrealistic goals—not too many friends, books, hobbies, concerts, movies, walks, volunteer jobs—trying to prove ourselves. We may tire more easily than we used to, and fatigue reduces pleasure and can bring on depression. We must watch over our dwindling budget carefully—impulse buying is not for most of us. Many goods and services are free or low in cost for older people. We must watch for, and take advantage of, them.

If a woman is retired, she might do well to return to, or develop, a hobby or craft that interests her—art, music, sewing, knitting, embroidery. (Watching TV can be more rewarding and less guilt-making if one's hands are busy.) Many newly retired women join an organized group with interests like their own, be it for self-development or social service or political advocacy. Adult continuing education classes are inexpensive and rewarding.

Some social scientists tell us that pets can lessen loneliness in older people. If one chooses to have a pet (which might be only if a person has had and enjoyed one previously), it must be remembered that animals have rights and needs, too. They can't be left alone very long. They must be watered, fed, and tended (dogs must be walked; cats need litter boxes if they stay indoors; birds need clean cages, fish clean tanks). And animals' life spans are not very long, and the loss of a loved pet can be almost the last straw.

Some thoughts for a typical day by ourselves, for ourselves:

Waking and getting up can be difficult for older

people. Take it easily and slowly and, if your physical health allows, stretch, bend, and rotate arms, legs, back, head, hands, and feet as you arise to get circulation going and ease stiffness.

Get ready for the day early. Staying in bed or in a robe too long can be demoralizing.

Use the media—newspapers, periodicals, radio, TV—to stay abreast of world doings.

Call, or write someone during the day to keep in touch.

Exercise and eat properly. If possible, go outdoors at least once, and breathe deeply wherever you are.

Do something useful, something pleasurable, and something healthful at least once a day. You will feel better for it.

Get enough rest but not too much. Keep moving.

To Help Us Help Ourselves

Such groups as the widow-to-widow programs, Alcoholics Anonymous, and single-purpose organizations for people suffering from a specific disease have shown that few if any can help a person through or with a crisis as well as others who have been or are still there. Because this is so, older people may be able to understand and help each other with the problems of aging better than some of those who have not yet arrived.

To strengthen existing friend-to-friend and neighbor-to-neighbor support, we older women might think about organizing informal mutual/self-help groups. Such organizations could not only provide needed services to add to those already at hand but could also expand human contacts by helping their members feel needed and belonging and by creating opportunities to learn new skills and assume new roles. Such a group might grow from an already existing setting or function—geographical (neighbors), social (card players, senior center activities), caregiving (Foster Grandparents, volunteer hospital services), or just old friendships.

When a mutual/self-help group is formed or identifies itself, it might define the concrete needs of its members and possibly, as it expands, the needs of its community. It could provide such services as visiting homebound members; regular checks by telephone; raised blinds and other signals to ensure that no member is in trouble; help such as grocery shopping, light housekeeping, plant and pet tending when a member is temporarily indisposed; transportation and company to health care facilities; neighborhood house watches. Chore exchanges answer some basic personal needs. (Anyone at any age who lives alone is at some risk.)

As a group's activities become established and members feel themselves to be effective, it might expand its work into more formal community programs such as car pooling and blood pressure checks and finally, in cooperation with other community organizations, nutrition projects, health maintenance centers, and home repair and transportation services.

The impetus behind mutual/self-help groups varies. Sometimes a professional sponsor, a community mental health center or a government aging program, seeing a need, will initiate a mutual/self-help group, but in most cases a group's beginnings are spontaneously based on shared needs. As the group evolves, leaders, who are usually "natural helpers," may need to be trained in organizational and teaching skills by professionals. These "experts" should take care, however, to serve only as catalyst/consultants and should withdraw as soon as they are no longer needed. (For instance, this Guide was developed as a part of NYU's Older Woman's Health Project and was used as a text during the last stage of the project, when older women were trained to become leaders of workshops on mental and physical wellness. It is hoped that the network will reach out to other communities throughout the nation. The project also plans to provide connections with other organizations concerned with older women's health.)

A mutual/self-help group will need to be minimally funded through its own efforts—rummage sales, social events, raffles—and it will need to be sustained through a sound and flexible organizational structure so that its programs will continue as long as they are needed.

There is strength in numbers, and some older people might do well to organize to help others help themselves.

To Remain or Become Involved—Advocacy

Although people are said to disengage as they grow older, we older people should continue to cherish our established relationships and create new ones. Chapter 5 of this book discusses problems and solutions involving our personal relationships. In this section, we are concerned with involvement in public causes and issues, particularly those related to women and older people.

A situation which is new, very important, and a little awesome has entered the lives of older people and older women in particular in the past decade—real political power.

In her recent book, *The Second Stage*, Betty Friedan writes, "That immutable, overshadowing definition of women as breeders of the race, once rooted in biological, historical necessity, only became a mystique, a defense against reality, as it denied the possibilities and necessities of growth opened by women's new life span in advanced technological society." In other words, we older women are the statistical force behind today's great feminist movement. Heady stuff, indeed!

In today's world a woman's last child may have left home before she is 50; if she has reached 65, she can expect to live an additional 17.5 years. Her voting record is excellent. With a voting power of 13 million people, 90 percent of whom are registered and most of whom vote regularly, we older women represent a large and growing political body. Unhappily, the majority of older women in the 1980s do not understand the uses of this political power. This will change as our better-educated and less socially oppressed sisters reach olderhood, but in the meantime it will pay today's older women to become politically aware in order to help ourselves and our cohorts.

R. N. Butler writes in *Aging and Mental Health* that:

> The potential strength of the elderly is likely to prove to be one of the "sleeper" surprises of future politics. Almost 90% are registered to vote and two-thirds vote regularly, many more than in any other age group. It remains for older people to organize themselves for political action and influence. There is even now a growing restlessness and militance among the elderly for "senior power." . . . Along with political strength can come a new sense of self-respect and a respect from others that will not be dependent on solicitude but will be a sober recognition of power at the ballot box on public issues.

About women and political power, he adds:

> A considerable number of older women have forged unique positions for themselves in terms of identity, personal achievement, and even financial and political power, but they need to be located and made visible.

How does one become involved in social and

political action?

1. Be or become an informed voter. This may take a lot of doing: reading and listening to news and pinpointing issues concerning women and older people, such as Social Security, Medicare, Medicaid, nursing home reform, housing, access to health care, pension rights, displaced homemakers, nuclear proliferation and pollution, and funding programs.
2. Discover and join local political action groups or chapters of national organizations. If you are already involved with a religious and/or community organization, find out how it might serve your advocacy goals. Think of how related organizations in your community might work together toward common goals.
3. Attend meetings regularly and urge your friends to join you.
4. Keep in touch with your elected representatives.
5. Consider running for elective office. Older women can get themselves elected to office in states where they live in large numbers, and many have time to lobby, campaign, and promote candidates.
6. Contribute money (if you can spare it) to your causes. (Women are reputed to control more than half of the nation's wealth.)

We older women must make certain that, individually and together, we do *not* remain the most oppressed sector of our society—isolated, sick, poor, and invisible—but rather become physically and economically improved, socially respected, and politically outspoken.

FOUR

Health
Problems

COMMUNICATING WITH THE HEALTH CARE SYSTEM

What Do You Expect at Your Age?

The answer should be, "the same quality of care that is afforded to anyone in this technologically advanced society." Unfortunately, our experience and most of the experiences described in a nationally distributed questionnaire do not bear out this statement. The question read, "Do you want to share any experiences that you have had with the health care system?" A sampling of our respondents replied:

> "It is very unresponsive to anything but discrete pathologies. It has no interest in prevention. It assumes that if you are over 50, you are ready for the nursing home and anything the matter with you 'is to be expected at your age.' It is no good!"

> "The need to raise consciousness [of all women] to the fact that health care is just one of many areas where *females* receive disparate treatment. Also that health care is a feminism

consumer issue."

"I do not feel the health care system accords older persons appropriate respect. I do not think an older person should be called by her first name, for instance, by someone she has never previously met (clerks, nurses, etc.). I do not feel that an older person should be 'patronized.' I have noticed this in reference to my husband especially. Even if one is confused or dizzy momentarily, this does not mean that she cannot assume responsibility, nor that she doesn't have a right to express doubts and reservations."

"I followed a doctor's advice and tried nursing home care [for her mother]. Nightmare! Our greatest national disgrace!"

"Nothing out of the ordinary. I have been treated as a nonperson, with boundless time to wait, as have most other women patients."

"Now I am 60 years old and while I have been a healthy person there are times I would like to find a few simple answers to a question instead of 'it's your age.'"

"I've avoided it so far." (The most damning of all.)

Today, many of the disabilities long thought to be associated with aging are actually symptoms of treatable disease. The health care practitioner's often heard response to an older person's physical complaints (as quoted by our respondents), "What do you expect at your age?" no longer has any credence.

As we have seen, many older women are largely displeased with today's health care delivery, and steps are being taken at governmental and institutional levels to improve the situation. Health care practitioners of the caliber of Robert Butler, author of the Pulitzer Prize-winning book *Why Survive? Being Old in America*, have taken up the cry with many voices, but it is primarily up to us, the consumers, to effect the necessary changes, and we can do this only by becoming *educated* consumers.

What does being educated about health care involve? First, as discussed in Chapter 2, "Maintaining Wellness," it means knowing our own bodies. If we are sufficiently and objectively aware of our own normal bodily functions, we can probably detect persistent variations from this norm and will seek medical help promptly.

Second, we must be familiar with the "system." Whence comes this help? Again, if we have followed the guidelines for maintaining wellness, we have had regular general physical checkups, as well as GYN, dental, and eye examinations and, therefore, have an appropriate health care practitioner at hand. However, when we seek help for a physical abnormality, we should be prepared to ask the appropriate questions and fully understand the answers.

These are some suggestions for a first visit:

1. Write down your symptoms as you perceive

them and the questions you want to ask.

2. Remember that you have the legal right to bring another person with you.
3. Report your symptoms as accurately as possible.
4. Report all prescriptive and over-the-counter medications you are taking.
5. If you don't understand the health care practitioner's language, request a simpler explanation (you are not the person with specialized training).
6. If you are not satisfied with the results of your visit, get another opinion. *Always* get at least a second opinion when surgery is recommended.

After the health care practitioner has completed all aspects of the examination, including tests and referrals, ask for the diagnosis (nature of the disease) as far as the health care practitioner can tell, the prognosis (the probable outcome), and the prescribed treatment. Questions regarding these three factors should be answered honestly, understandably (without condescension), and unhurriedly.

You should know: what the condition is called; its bodily symptoms; the probable outcome following treatment; recommended treatment or procedure, how performed, by whom, how often, and how prolonged; where (in hospital, outpatient clinic, office); amount of pain; conditions of recuperation; possible side effects or complications; how to prevent recurrence; alternatives to surgery, if recommended (here again a second opinion is always advisable—you may even want a third opinion); prescribed medication, dosage, side effects, restrictions; nature of treatment, accepted or experimental; estimated cost of treatment; and insurance coverage.

"Informed consent" is your right, as consumers of health care. Receive sufficient information about the treatment prescribed before you agree to it. It is also your right to be heard and respected by health care providers. You are a person, not a disease.

This chapter is not intended as a tool for self-diagnosis but rather as a guide to some common health problems of older women. It is designed to help you become educated and self-respecting consumers of health care.

SPECIFIC HEALTH PROBLEMS OF OLDER WOMEN

Alcoholism and Alcohol Abuse

"In old age few things break up a person faster than alcohol," writes Alex Comfort in *A Good Age*. The degree or even presence of this devastation depends, of course, on the way alcohol is handled by an older person. As a matter of fact, many professionals concerned with aging recommend an occasional or even a regular glass of wine for stimulation or a change of pace. However, alcohol is an addictive drug and a depressant that, if used unwisely, can dramatically compound the physical, emotional, and social problems of aging.

There is an ongoing controversy among medical and social service professionals as to what "alcoholism" is and who an "alcoholic" is. In the 1950s the World Health Organization and the American Medical Association declared alcoholism a disease, raising the issue as to whether personal responsibility plays any role in alcohol addiction. However this may be, if a person finds that she can no longer do without or control her drinking, or that her drinking habits are changing, she has a problem and should take immediate steps to solve it.

Confirmed alcoholics (mostly males) do survive into old age and will probably continue their addiction, risking serious, irreversible, and often fatal degenerative conditions. More relevant to the purpose of this book are older people who become alcoholics only in later life.

Having failed to cope with the stresses of growing older by maintaining their physical and mental well-being and adapting to change, they turn to alcohol as a crutch. Some become alcoholics to relieve boredom; others, to cope with the pain of losing loved ones. Many are "beginning" drinkers; others, occasional, social, or habitual but controlled drinkers who become seriously addicted as they grow older. However, drinking leads to new and more severe problems. These problems are often compounded for an older woman because, ashamed of her addiction, she may drink only secretly and alone. Becoming more isolated and depressed, she may neglect her personal needs, alienate her family and friends, and become a lonely and unwilling slave to alcohol. Not a pretty picture! Indeed, alcoholism is one of the ugliest of human conditions.

There are approximately 10 million alcoholics in the United States; 4 million of these are women. It is not known exactly how many of these women are over 55. However, reports indicate that 10 to 20 percent of nursing home residents are alcoholics and that possibly 20 percent of people over 50 have a drinking problem. (Widowers over 65 appear to have the highest rates.)

At this time we do not know what causes alcoholism. There may be an inherited tendency to the illness. Psychological stress certainly contributes to its development, but whether certain personality types are more prone to alcoholism is unclear. Social and cultural factors such as alcohol use and importance within ethnic groups and a view of drinking as desirable adult behavior also affect alcohol abuse.

Alcohol has a variety of undesirable effects on the body. Since alcohol contains calories but virtually no other nutrients, heavy drinkers can suffer from malnutrition. As little as four to five drinks per day can cause liver damage due to fat buildup in that organ. Prolonged alcohol abuse has more serious effects, including alcoholic hepatitis, cirrhosis of the liver, disorders of the nervous system, brain damage, low blood sugar, and a serious form of heart disease. Alcoholics have higher-than-average rates of peptic ulcer; pancreatitis; gastritis; and cancer of the mouth, throat, esophagus, larynx, and liver.

Among diabetics, alcohol consumption may increase blood sugar levels and make diabetes more difficult to control.

Alcohol and many medications do not mix. The effects of tranquilizers, sleeping pills, narcotics, and medications for anxiety and depression are intensified by alcohol, and could lead to coma and even death. Alcohol also reacts unfavorably with antihistamines; drugs which prevent blood from clotting (like Coumadin); some blood pressure medications such as Aldomet, Lasix, and Reserpine; and oral medications for diabetes. In addition, alcohol is present in many over-the-counter drugs such as cough syrups and elixirs. When taking any medication it is important to check whether alcohol will interfere with its action; the content labels on all over-the-counter medications should also be checked.

Alcoholics Anonymous (AA), the worldwide self-help organization, has outlined steps toward the rehabilitation of an alcoholic. The first and most difficult step, because it must be taken alone, is to admit that alcohol is controlling one's life: to state unequivocally and openly: "I am an alcoholic." The second is to stop drinking. This step usually requires help of some kind. If a person is physically addicted, hospitalization for detoxification ("drying out") may be indicated. A local chapter of the National Council on Alcoholism can provide information about detoxification centers.

Following this, many treatment programs are available to help a person stay sober, of which AA is probably the best known and singly most effective. Sometimes membership in AA or other self-help groups is combined with professional therapy to alleviate the basic causes of the addiction. Some alcoholics take a daily dose of disulfiram (Antabuse), which can cause headaches, nausea, vomiting, dizziness, and chest pain if alcohol is ingested.

AA members in good standing are people who believe that they cannot handle alcohol and no longer drink it at all. They provide strong individual and group support for those who genuinely want to stop drinking even though the path to sobriety may have many turnings. Their patience is legion. They understand because they have been there.

Al-Anon, an affiliated organization, provides information and counseling to friends and relatives of alcoholics. Information about AA and Al-Anon can be found in the telephone directory in almost any city in the world.

Arthritis

Arthritis is not one disease but many—there are over one hundred different kinds. Some type of arthritis affects 50 million Americans.

The word "arthritis" literally means "inflammation of the joints." However, it is used today to describe conditions causing aches and pains but not necessarily inflammation (warmth, redness, tenderness, swelling) of joints and connective tissue. Some of the more common types of arthritis are osteoarthritis, rheumatoid arthritis, gout, ankylosis spondylitis, and rheumatic fever. In this section we will discuss osteoarthritis, the most common form and the one most likely to occur among older women.

OSTEOARTHRITIS:

Osteoarthritis is considered a disease of older people, although it can occur at any age. Sixteen million Americans have symptoms of this illness, which is also called degenerative joint disease (DJD). Another 30 million have no symptoms but have changes due to osteoarthritis detected by x-ray. The incidence of osteoarthritis does increase with age. In fact, 97 percent of those over 60 have some evidence of the illness. Overall, women are affected twice as often as are men. Many experts think that everyone will develop osteoarthritis eventually if she or he simply lives long enough.

Osteoarthritis is often called the "wear-and-tear" disease. It involves the cartilage, the tough gristle at the end of bones which acts as a cushion to enable the joint to operate smoothly. Over the years this cartilage can become soft, frayed, lose its elasticity, and even wear away. Therefore, the joint cannot operate smoothly and may become painful and stiff. There is usually little or no inflammation, however.

The cause of osteoarthritis is not really known. Both heredity and obesity seem to affect its development. There is also some evidence that a joint which is injured or repeatedly abused is more prone to develop osteoarthritis. However, no one knows why some people have severe osteoarthritis at an

142

early age while others escape relatively unscathed even though there is x-ray evidence that they have the disease.

Osteoarthritis can be divided into two types. One type involves the joints of the fingers and toes. These joints become enlarged, and bony growths called Heberden's and Bouchard's nodes often develop there. There may be some pain and stiffness, but the major problem is cosmetic (the disfigurement of these joints).

The other type affects the major weight-bearing joints—knees and hips as well as the spine. Some experts consider osteoarthritis of the spine to be a separate type. Interestingly, osteoarthritis rarely affects the ankle, which is certainly a weight-bearing joint. Osteoarthritis of the spine seldom causes symptoms unless there is pressure on a nerve in the back. On the other hand, osteoarthritis of the hip or knee often causes pain and stiffness and limits mobility of the affected joint, which may make walking difficult.

SYMPTOMS:

As we have noted, osteoarthritis often has no symptoms. If they do occur, they usually include pain and stiffness, most severe in the morning, and decreased mobility of the involved joint. Symptoms may be worse in bad weather. Rarely is there inflammation (redness, warmth, tenderness, swelling). There are no generalized body changes such as weakness, malaise, weight loss, or fever. Osteoarthritis does not affect any organs.

DIAGNOSIS:

Diagnosis is made by physical examination. X-rays are useful, since osteoarthritis shows characteristic changes in the joints. A blood test called a "sedimentation rate," which is normal in osteoarthritis but elevated in other forms of arthritis, may be performed.

Your regular health care practitioner can usually diagnose and treat osteoarthritis. However, you may also want to consult a rheumatologist, a physician who specializes in the diagnosis and treatment of all types of arthritis.

TREATMENT:

The goals of treatment are to maintain and/or improve joint function, relieve symptoms, and prevent further deterioration. Treatment generally consists of a regular exercise program balanced with rest, weight reduction if overweight, and application of heat to the affected area. Medication may be useful but is less important than other kinds of treatment.

A regular exercise program usually combines some type of regular physical activity—walking or swimming seem to be best—with special calisthenic exercises to put the affected joint through its full range of motion. Your health care practitioner will prescribe the specific exercises which will be most helpful to you. Exercise helps maintain joint function while making bones and joint-supporting ligaments and muscles stronger, helps in weight maintenance or reduction, and aids relaxation. When starting an exercise program, proceed slowly and gradually and build up your strength and endurance. Severe pain is a signal to stop. Mild pain is not. Listen to your body. Many people find a warm bath or shower, hot washcloths or a heating pad useful before exercise to improve mobility and reduce pain in the affected joints.

The best diet for osteoarthritis is a balanced, nutritious one which maintains health and normal weight. There is no special diet which prevents or cures any form of arthritis. Fad diets or large doses of vitamins, minerals, hormones, or other supplements have not been shown to have any positive effects on arthritis. In addition, they may be dangerous to your health as well as a drain on your pocketbook.

In severe cases of osteoarthritis of a weight-bearing joint, surgery may be a treatment option. Total hip replacement and total knee replacement surgery are major advances in the treatment of osteoarthritis with a high success rate and minimal risk for most people. This surgery usually provides total pain relief and the ability to walk normally and to return to normal activities.

Unfortunately, many people think that arthritis signals the end of their ability to have sexual relations. However, sexual activity may actually help relieve arthritis symptoms.

MEDICATION:
Many people are surprised to learn that *aspirin* is the drug of choice in treating osteoarthritis. So many of us take aspirin for any minor complaint

without a second thought that we are amazed to learn that it is an important and powerful drug with many effects on the body. For pain relief, aspirin is taken in small or moderate doses, usually two five-grain tablets every four hours as needed. If aspirin is used to suppress inflammation (not usually the case in osteoarthritis), it is taken in much higher doses. Since aspirin can interfere with blood clotting and with other medications, and may have side effects, self-treatment of osteoarthritis is not advisable. Follow the advice of your health care practitioner.

The most common side affects of aspirin are nausea and stomach upset and, in higher doses, ringing in the ears. To control nausea or stomach problems, your health care practitioner may suggest that you take aspirin after meals, after taking an antacid such as Maalox or Gelusil, or switch to coated aspirin (such as Ecotrin), which dissolves in the intestine rather than in the stomach.

Unless your health care practitioner recommends a specific type of aspirin, the best aspirin to buy is the cheapest, plain, store-brand aspirin in five-grain tablets. Brand names contain the same amount of aspirin for a much higher price. Be sure to read labels, and beware of gimmicks like "extra strength" and "arthritis aspirin." These are usually just two or three aspirins combined into one tablet or capsule at several times the price of regular aspirin. Avoid aspirin containing other ingredients such as caffeine, phenacetin, or antihistamines. You don't need the extra medication or the extra cost.

A non-aspirin-containing pain reliever such as acetaminophen (Tylenol, Datril, and others) may be recommended for those people who cannot tolerate aspirin. Acetaminophen is a mild pain reliever which does not usually cause nausea or stomach upset. It has some effect on inflammation.

Several other medications which are sometimes used to treat osteoarthritis can be grouped together into a category called "nonsteroidal anti-inflammatory drugs" (NSAID). They are so called because they are not steroids as are cortisone and prednisone, but they do decrease inflammation as do cortisone, prednisone, and aspirin. As a group, they tend to be mildly effective in reducing pain but are used primarily for their anti-inflammatory properties. They are substantially more expensive than aspirin; however, they may be better tolerated than aspirin by some people. They are not equally effective for each person—you may have to try several to find the one that is most effective for you. Side effects include stomach irritation, nausea, heartburn, indigestion, and, with Butazolidin, a serious blood problem called aplastic anemia. Although great claims have been made for many of these medications, with heavy promotion and advertising by individual drug companies, they are not miracle drugs. Aspirin remains the drug of choice to treat osteoarthritis. (Examples of NSAID include Butazolidin, Indocin, Nalfon, Motrin, Naprosyn, Clinoril, and Tolectin.)

Medications such as steroids, gold salts, and penicillamine are used to treat forms of arthritis other than osteoarthritis.

Many experts feel that the development of osteoarthritis can be delayed or minimized by following a regular exercise program. Using bones and joints regularly makes them, as well as the surrounding ligaments and muscles, stronger while nourishing the joint cartilage. Experts also recommend maintaining a normal weight because overweight places extra stress on bones and joints. Good posture also reduces stress on joints. In addition, it is just common sense to warm up muscles and joints before performing strenuous activities, and to wear the correct kind of shoes, properly fitted, for whatever activity you are about to undertake.

Cancer

Despite the fact that heart disease is the leading cause of death among older people, cancer is the most feared disease. It has a reputation for being a hopeless, fatal disease even though many cancers can be cured if detected early enough.

Cancer is not a homogeneous disease. It is a group of diseases with many different causes. Some of these causes, such as cigarette smoking or exposure to cancer-causing chemicals, are avoidable. Therefore, it is important to be aware of what is known about the causes, detection, and treatment of cancer so that you can decrease your risk of developing it.

BREAST CANCER:

Breast cancer is the most frequent cancer among women. The chances of the average woman developing breast cancer are one in eleven. Furthermore, three groups have a higher-than-average risk of developing breast cancer. These are women over age 50, women whose mother or sisters have had breast cancer, and women who have already had breast cancer. Other factors which may increase the risk are long-term cystic disease of the breast, onset of menstruation before age 11, having no children or having a first pregnancy after age 30, high-fat diet, upper socioeconomic class, and being a white person.

The specific cause of breast cancer is unkown. However, the earlier the cancer is detected and treated, the better the chance is for its cure.

It is reassuring to know that eight out of ten breast lumps are not cancer. However, any lump, thickening, skin dimpling or puckering, or nipple discharge should be examined and evaluated by your health care practitioner as soon as possible. Fear of breast cancer prevents some women from doing so. This is unfortunate, causing unnecessary anxiety for the large majority who do not have cancer and delaying effective treatment for those who do.

Since 90 percent of breast lumps are discovered by women themselves, early detection begins with breast self-examination (BSE). All women should examine their breasts once a month. Women past menopause should pick a date they will remember, such as the first of the month or the monthly anniversary of their birth dates to remind themselves to do a BSE. The examination is performed monthly so that women become familiar with the appearance and texture of their own breasts, enabling them to recognize a change.

In addition to a monthly BSE, all women should have their breasts examined yearly by their health care practitioners. This can be done during the yearly gynecological examination or routine physical examination.

The third method of detection is mammography. This consists of special x-rays of the breasts which can reveal tumors which are too small to be found by breast examination. The American Cancer Society recommends a yearly mammogram for women over 50. Other experts recommend mammography at regular intervals but not necessarily once a year. Mammography has been controversial because of the possibility that radiation from the x-rays themselves may cause cancer. However, with current x-ray equipment the dose of radiation is quite small, and for women over 50 it is thought that the value of the examination outweighs the risk.

Two other detection methods, which are still under investigation, are thermography, in which special film records heat patterns of the breast, and ultrasound, which bounces sound waves off the breast tissue. Neither of these techniques use x-rays, so there is no chance of radiation exposure.

If a breast lump is found, a biopsy is usually performed to establish a diagnosis. If cancer is present, there are now several options to the once standard radical mastectomy (surgical removal of the breast, surrounding lymph nodes, and muscle). Studies are under way to evaluate less disfiguring surgery such as removal of the tumor only (lumpectomy), or breast only, along with follow-up treatment with radiation to kill any remaining cancer cells. If the breast is removed, breast reconstructive surgery is now available.

Since there are so many choices, it is important to discuss all available alternatives with your health care practitioner and surgeon. In the past few years women have demanded and obtained many changes in the treatment of breast cancer. It is up to you to take advantage of them.

CANCER OF THE UTERUS AND OVARIES:

There are two types of uterine cancer: cancer of the cervix (the neck of the uterus situated at the end of the vagina) and cancer of the lining of the uterus itself. The rate of cervical cancer decreases after age 60. It is highly curable and is diagnosed by a pap smear, recommended for all women on a regular basis.

Cancer of the lining of the uterus (endometrial cancer) occurs most often in women over 50. It is more common in women who are obese, have a late menopause, have never had children, have high blood presssure or diabetes, and who are receiving oral estrogen therapy. This type of cancer may not be detected by a pap smear.

The main warning sign of both of these cancers

is vaginal bleeding after menopause. The diagnosis is usually made by biopsy. Treatment for both types is surgery and/or radiation therapy.

The incidence of cancer of the ovaries increases with age. It is known as a silent cancer, since, unfortunately, there are very few signs and symptoms of this disease until it is well established. Abdominal discomfort, gas, or bloating are often the only symptoms. Examination of the ovaries by palpation during the pelvic examination should be part of every woman's yearly gynecological examination. Ovarian cancer is treated with surgery and medication (chemotherapy).

ESTROGEN REPLACEMENT THERAPY:

Estrogen replacement therapy (ERT) has been used to treat menopausal symptoms such as hot flashes and to prevent and treat osteoporosis (a disease of older people in which bones become more fragile and fracture easily). Unfortunately, oral estrogen therapy also increases the risk of endometrial cancer. The risk of developing this cancer increases the higher the dose and the longer the estrogen is taken. However, recent studies have suggested that adding progesterone (another female hormone) at times during the treatment cycle may actually decrease the risk of developing this cancer.

Women for whom estrogen therapy is recommended should thoroughly discuss the risks and benefits of this treatment with their health care practitioners. Women who are taking replacement estrogen should have a pelvic examination every six months as well as a biopsy of the lining of the uterus at frequent intervals.

CANCER OF THE COLON:

This is the second most common cancer among both women and men. Signs and symptoms include rectal bleeding, a change in bowel habits, weight loss, black or bloody bowel movements, chronic constipation, weakness, and anemia. It is now thought that high consumption of red meat and a diet which is low in fiber are related to the development of colon cancer. (See the section on fiber in Chapter 2.) Therefore, increasing fiber in the diet along with adequate fluid intake and avoiding chronic constipation may reduce the risk. Since early detection is most important, a yearly rectal examination is recommended. An annual sigmoidoscopy may be recommended in some cases.

LUNG CANCER:

Lung cancer is a largely preventable cancer, since cigarette smoking is its primary cause. Unfortunately, lung cancer rates are rising among women. Detection is difficult until the cancer is well established, and the success of surgical treatment is limited. The best way to prevent lung cancer is to stop smoking.

Depression

Depression is a state of being which defies definition. It may be a normal or abnormal mood state and range from a transient unpleasant feeling to a serious psychiatric illness. All of us become depressed at times, but feeling depressed means different things to different people. It has been described as sadness, loneliness, boredom, apathy, despair, dejection, and numbness. It is normal for feelings like this to occur in people who are not psychiatrically ill. However, if these feelings persist for long periods of time and prevent an individual from carrying out normal activities, it is wise to obtain professional help.

Depression is said to be common among older people, although statistics are difficult to obtain. (There have been very few studies of depression in people over age 55.) It is unclear whether the incidence of depression is about equal for both sexes after age 55 or whether more women are diagnosed as depressed simply because they are more likely to seek professional help. In any event, there are a number of life changes and stresses which can produce depression in older women. These include the losses which occur as one ages, such as loss of family and friends through death or distance and loss of health, employment, independence, and productivity. Other stresses include widowhood, lack of money, social and cultural isolation, and role change as one ages. Such illnesses as influenza or heart attacks and certain medications used in the treatment of high blood pressure can also cause depression.

The difference between normal grief or sadness and depression which requires treatment is one of degree. Common signs and symptoms are weight loss, decreased appetite, apathy, insomnia, fatigue, loss of sex drive, indecisiveness, irritability, and inability to concentrate. In an older person depression can be masked by a physical illness or can be confused with senility. Tragically, there are people who are labeled as "senile" who are actually suffering from depression, a treatable illness.

Treatment of depression varies with the type of illness. *Reactive* depression (usually a short-term illness with a clearly defined cause) responds best to psychotherapy by a qualified professional. Drugs are not usually used.

On the other hand, *endogenous* depression (usually a long-term depression with no clear-cut cause and more intense symptoms) is treated with antidepressant drug therapy or with electroconvulsive therapy (ECT).

The medications used to treat this type of depression are called tricyclic antidepressants (examples are Elavil, Triavil, and others). Many experts are concerned about the use of these drugs by people over age 65, since there has been little research on the effects of these drugs on this age group. Although these medications can be quite helpful in the treatment of depression, they have a number of side effects which can prevent or limit their use among older people. For example, they may cause drowsiness, constipation, urinary retention, or a sudden drop in blood pressure upon standing. They interfere with the action of medications for high blood pressure. In addition, the effect of these drugs is intensified by drinking alcohol. It usually takes from one to three weeks for the medication to take effect. Older people require a smaller dose than do others.

After years of disrepute in some circles, ECT has become a much safer and more acceptable form of treatment for certain types of depression. With improved methods of treatment, problems such as memory loss after ECT have been reduced. If it is recommended, it is an alternative that should at least be given consideration.

Eye Problems

CATARACTS:

Cataract formation is the most common eye problem among older people; it is present to some degree in at least 95 percent of those over age 65. A cataract is a clouding of the normally transparent lens which is situated in the eye behind the iris and the pupil. The lens works on the same principle as the lens of a camera, focusing a picture of what we see on the back of the eye. There the image can be transmitted to, and interpreted by, the brain. After age 40, the lens becomes less elastic and takes on a yellowish color. These changes interfere with the passage of light through the lens, causing the blurred vision which is the main symptom of a cataract forming. Usually there is neither pain nor other symptoms.

At this time, we do not know how to prevent or slow down cataract formation in older people. The only effective treatment at present is surgical removal, which is successful in 95 to 98 percent of cases. When blurred vision interferes with normal activities, surgery is usually indicated. Sometimes a cataract must be removed because another eye disease is present. Very early cataracts which do not significantly interfere with vision do not have to be removed but should be examined periodically by an ophthalmologist (eye specialist) or primary health care practitioner.

Sophisticated surgical techniques and local anesthesia have made cataract removal increasingly safe and effective, resulting in shorter hospital stays and quicker recovery than in the past. However, as with any surgery, there are risks of infection, bleeding, and other complications. Fortunately, in cataract surgery such risks are very small.

Since the lens of the eye is being removed during this surgery, some other way of focusing light inside the eye is necessary. The three methods currently used are glasses, contact lenses, and artificial lens implants (intraocular lenses, or IOL).

The glasses used are quite thick and powerful, enlarging the size of objects viewed through them by one-third. If they are used to correct vision in only one eye, they will cause double vision (the normal eye will continue to see objects at normal size).

This problem of double vision can be minimized by the use of a contact lens in the affected eye, because a contact lens comes closer to replacing the removed lens. It is well tolerated by many people; however, not everyone has the dexterity required to insert and remove the lens. This problem has been alleviated somewhat by the recent development of "extended-wear" contact lenses which usually require removal and cleaning only once a month.

The third method, still relatively new and controversial, is the insertion of an artificial plastic lens into the eye. This has the advantage of restoring vision in the affected eye to what it was before the cataract appeared without the distortion of glasses or the bother of contact lenses. However, the plastic lens is a foreign object in the eye; it may not be well tolerated and may have unknown long-term side effects. Artificial lenses are not used in those people who have other eye diseases or who have only one eye.

You should thoroughly discuss the advantages and disadvantages of each of these methods with your ophthalmologist in order to decide which is best for you.

GLAUCOMA:

Glaucoma is an increase in pressure within the eye which, if not treated, damages the nerve responsible for vision (the optic nerve). It is the third leading cause of blindness in the United States. Glaucoma, which can be successfully treated if diagnosed in time, is primarily a disease of people over 40. Although the cause of the disease is often not known, it may result from eye injury, infection, cataracts or other eye diseases, and some medications.

Unfortunately, the most common form of glaucoma (chronic glaucoma) has no symptoms, and those who have it may be unaware of its presence until visual loss occurs. Therefore, early diagnosis is most important. Experts recommend that those over age 40 have their eyes checked for increased pressure every one to two years by an ophthalmologist or at a health screening clinic. People with a family or personal history of glaucoma or other serious eye disease usually require more frequent examinations.

There is also an acute form of glaucoma which is relatively rare but is a medical emergency, since permanent loss of vision can occur within hours. Fortunately, this type of glaucoma has symptoms. These may include severe eye and facial pain, nausea and vomiting, decreased or blurred vision with haloes or rainbows around lights, and redness of the eye. If you have these symptoms, you should see an ophthalmologist at once.

TREATMENT:

Chronic glaucoma, the most common type, is usually successfully treated with medication. Eye drops such as pilocarpine, Epinephrine, or timolol are the treatment of choice. These decrease the pressure within the eye by improving the eye's drainage system or decreasing the amount of fluid produced. (These fluids are within the eye and have nothing to do with tears or other external fluids.) These eye drops are usually well tolerated, although they may cause some blurring of vision. Most eye drops must be inserted several times daily.

There is also a time-release medication called

Ocusert which is inserted in the eye once a week and which allows medication to be released at a steady rate. The major problem with this medication is its cost, which is several times higher than that of most eye drops.

Oral medication, such as Diamox, may also be used, usually in combination with eye drops. Since Diamox may have serious side effects such as kidney stones, weakness, weight loss, and depression, it is usually used only in those people for whom eye drops alone are not effective.

Since chronic glaucoma has no symptoms, many people do not realize the seriousness of the disease and are unwilling to take their medication regularly or to spend money for it. Glaucoma causes permanent blindness if not treated. Regular use of eye drops or other medication is a small price to pay for the ability to see.

Treatment with medication is successful in most cases. However, if it is not effective, surgery is necessary to prevent visual loss. Fortunately, surgery for glaucoma has a very high success rate and carries a low risk.

Acute glaucoma almost always requires surgery to prevent a recurrence of symptoms, although eye drops and oral medication are usually used initially.

Heart Disease

As has been mentioned, heart disease is the leading cause of death in the United States. (Cancer, by the way, is a very distant second, not first, as many people think). Among older people, heart disease accounts for more illness and death than any other condition.

The three major risk factors for heart disease are cigarette smoking, high blood pressure, and high blood levels of cholesterol. Other risk factors include obesity, sedentary living, stress, age, heredity, a history of diabetes, and race (blacks are at greater risk).

There are many different kinds of heart disease. Here we shall discuss three of the most common: heart attack, angina, and congestive heart failure.

HEART ATTACK:

A heart attack (myocardial infarction) occurs when part of the heart muscle dies because its blood supply has been cut off. This is usually due to a blood clot blocking an artery which supplies the heart, but it may also be caused by a temporary spasm of these arteries.

Symptoms of a heart attack include pressure and an aching or pain in the center of the chest which may spread to the shoulders, neck, jaw, arms, or back and which last for several minutes or more.

However, some older people do not have *severe* chest pain; it may feel like a bad case of "indigestion." Other symptoms which may be present are dizziness, fainting, nausea, breathlessness, and sweating.

Most heart attack deaths occur after age 65. Women are less likely to have heart attacks than are men; the risk for women increases after menopause, however. Blacks are at a greater risk because they are more likely to have high blood pressure.

If you have symptoms of a heart attack, you should seek emergency care immediately. Most hospitals are now equipped to provide emergency cardiac care on a twenty-four-hour basis. You should be aware of which hospitals near you provide this service.

Treatment consists of hospitalization for approximately two weeks with gradual resumption of daily activities. A rehabilitation, education, and exercise program is usually begun in the hospital and is continued when the individual returns home.

Cardiopulmonary resuscitation (CPR) is the first-aid treatment administered to heart attack victims and others whose heart and breathing have stopped. It is a combination of mouth-to-mouth breathing and chest compression which should be performed only by those who have been trained. Anyone can learn, however. Check with your local Heart Association or health clinic for training programs in your area.

ANGINA PECTORIS:

Angina is a brief but recurrent chest pain caused by an inadequate supply of blood (which carries oxygen) to part of the heart muscle. The decreased blood supply is usually caused by a narrowing of the coronary arteries because of atherosclerosis, a build-up of fatty deposits along the walls of the arteries. The pain is usually described as an ache, pressure, tightness, or burning in the center of the chest or behind the breastbone. It can be brought on by exercise or by exposure to cold, stress, emotional upset, or a heavy meal, and is relieved by rest. Some people also have shortness of breath and palpitations along with chest pain.

Angina is usually treated with nitroglycerin tablets which dissolve under the tongue. Nitroglycerin relaxes the walls of the blood vessels supplying the heart, allowing more blood and oxygen to reach the heart muscle. Nitroglycerin may be taken to prevent angina when a situation arises in which an anginal attack usually occurs. It is also taken to treat an attack which is occurring. The most common side effects of nitroglycerin are headache and flushing. Nitroglycerin tablets gradually lose their potency when exposed to air. Therefore, a container of nitroglycerin tablets which has been opened is good for only about two months. Nitroglycerin is also available as an ointment, or impregnated in a disposable pad. In this way it is applied directly to the skin, providing continuous pain relief.

Other medications used in treatment are a long-acting nitrite similar to nitroglycerin, isosorbide dinitrate (Isordil), and propanolol (Inderal), which reduce the amount of oxygen needed by the heart. Another way to ward off anginal attacks is to avoid the activity which brings about the angina if possible.

A controversial method of treating angina which has not been helped by medical treatment is coronary artery bypass surgery. In this procedure a vein graft is taken from the leg and is used to bypass the blocked coronary artery, thus providing the heart muscle with an adequate supply of blood and oxygen. At this time, the procedure is thought to be effective only when certain arteries are blocked. The costs and risks of surgery as well as the pain and disability involved must also be considered. While surgery may help some people with angina, it is not an appropriate treatment for everyone.

CONGESTIVE HEART FAILURE:

Congestive heart failure is a condition in which the heart muscle has been weakened and therefore cannot pump blood to the rest of the body effectively. It may be caused by high blood pressure, rheumatic heart disease, or atherosclerosis. Symptoms include shortness of breath; tiredness; swelling of the ankles, legs, and feet (edema); cough; rapid weight gain (from edema); and mental confusion.

Treatment depends on both the severity of symptoms and the underlying cause of the illness. Usual treatment consists of rest; a low-salt/sodium diet; diuretics (water pills); and digitalis, which strengthens the heart muscle.

PREVENTION:
1. Control high blood pressure, if present, and check yearly for high blood pressure if blood pressure is now within normal range.
2. Stop smoking.
3. Exercise regularly. Brisk walking or swim-

ming are good ways to maintain cardiac health.
4. Maintain ideal weight.
5. Cut down on animal fats, watch salt intake, eat a variety of foods—lean meats, poultry, fish, low-fat dairy products, whole grain breads and cereals, fresh fruits and vegetables.
6. Drink plenty of water.
7. Get enough rest and relaxation.
8. Reduce or control emotional stress.

Hypertension (High Blood Pressure)

Blood pressure is the pressure of the blood, pumped by the heart, against the walls of the arteries. When, for a variety of reasons, this pressure is elevated, the heart must work harder than normal to accomplish its task. As a result of this overwork the heart muscle may become enlarged. When blood pressure remains elevated for a prolonged period of time, damage to the heart and blood vessels may ensue. High blood pressure is one of the three major risk factors for heart disease. (The other two major risk factors are cigarette smoking and an elevated blood cholesterol.) High blood pressure also increases the risk of stroke and kidney disease.

High blood pressure is one of the most prevalent chronic diseases in the United States. Approximately 15 to 20 percent of all adults have it, although many of these people either do not know that they have high blood pressure or are receiving inadequate treatment. Rates of high blood pressure tend to rise with age, primarily affecting men over 35 and women over 45. The rate is also higher among blacks. High blood pressure is a major cause of premature death from heart disease and stroke.

MEASURING BLOOD PRESSURE:

Blood pressure is measured by a simple device called a "sphygmomanometer," which indicates the pressure as the heart muscle contracts (systolic, the higher number) and as it relaxes (diastolic, the lower number). Both measurements are important in determining diagnosis and treatment.

There are no set measurements that can be considered "normal." Blood pressures can vary significantly with age, sex, and in individuals. According to the American Heart Association, persons 50 years of age or younger should have measurements below 140/90; those over 50, below 160/95. No magic numbers can be considered normal or abnormal for everyone, however.

It is important to note that elevated blood pressure at any age poses a great threat of heart disease and stroke and that older people with lower blood pressures tend to live longer than those with higher pressures. Low blood pressure, on the other hand, is not usually a health problem except in extreme cases.

CAUSES:

The cause of high blood pressure is unknown in 90 to 95 percent of cases. The condition does not develop overnight but is usually characterized by a slow, progressive rise over a period of years. A specific cause for high blood pressure is determined in only 5 to 10 percent of cases, sometimes related to kidney disease or to imbalance of hormone secretion.

It is important to note that the term "hypertension" means blood pressure which is higher than normal. It does not mean "anxious" or "excitable" and does not relate to a specific personality type. Calm people can have high blood pressure, too!

RISK FACTORS:

Factors which increase the risk of developing high blood pressure include:

1. *Family history.* People whose parents (one or both) have high blood pressure are most prone to develop this illness.
2. *Obesity.* Studies have shown that obesity increases the risk of high blood pressure. Similarly, a reduction in weight is often accompanied by a reduction in blood pressure.
3. *Age.* Blood pressure tends to rise with age.
4. *Sex.* High blood pressure is more prevalent in men than in women. There have been some indications that women "tolerate" high blood pressure better than men; however, research results have clearly pointed out that elevated blood pressure at any age or in any person is a potent risk factor for heart disease and stroke.
5. *Elevated cholesterol levels in blood, cigarette smoking, and diabetes.* All are related to high

blood pressure regardless of age, sex, or race.

6. *Sodium/salt (high intake).* The average American diet, which is very high in sodium/salt, is considered an important factor in the development of high blood pressure. In some people, the kidneys are unable to remove excessive salt from the bloodstream, which increases the volume of blood circulating in the body, causing the heart to pump harder and blood pressure to rise.

7. *Race.* High blood pressure is more prevalent among blacks.

8. *Stressful life style.* This also appears to be a contributing factor in the development of high blood pressure.

In addition, blood pressure varies according to the time of day and the kind of activity in which a person is engaged. It is usually lowest just before awakening in the morning. Strenuous physical activity can increase the systolic blood pressure 60–80 points. Excitement, nervous tension, or fright can also raise the systolic blood pressure.

SYMPTOMS:

Because high blood pressure has no characteristic symptoms, it is sometimes called the "silent killer." Diagnosis of high blood pressure is usually made only through a physical examination. Therefore, it is important to have one's blood pressure checked yearly. However, headache present upon awakening in the morning and subsiding spontaneously after

168

several hours can occur in persons with high blood pressure. Other possible complaints are fatigue, dizziness, lightheadedness, and visual difficulties.

If high blood pressure is suspected, it should be confirmed on several different occasions rather than be based on one reading, since blood pressure varies from moment to moment and can be affected by emotions or the surrounding environment.

PREVENTION:

To help prevent high blood pressure:

1. *Decrease salt intake.* Moderate salt restriction has recently been shown to reverse hypertension in 85 percent of mild cases and in 51 percent of severe cases in a five-year Mayo Clinic trial in which a low-salt, low-calorie diet was the only therapy. (See the section on nutrition in Chapter 2 for suggestions on salt reduction.)
2. *Reduce weight if necessary.* Extra body weight causes the heart to work harder to pump the blood to the entire body. Weight loss has been shown to be closely related to reduction of blood pressure. (See the section later in this chapter on obesity and weight control.)
3. *Stop smoking.*
4. *Decrease intake of cholesterol and saturated fat.* An elevated blood cholesterol level is an important factor in the development of heart disease. (See the section on nutrition in Chapter 2 for suggestions.)

5. *Decrease stress.* Excess stress or tension due to emotional pressure causes the body to release chemicals such as adrenalin. Adrenalin increases the heartbeat and narrows the blood vessels. Both conditions contribute to high blood pressure. (See the section on stress in Chapter 2.)

6. *Exercise regularly.* Not only does regular exercise help in controlling weight and in shaping up the body, but physical conditioning may lower blood pressure. Exercise should be done regularly, and activity should be increased very gradually within your capability. If you have a physical condition that restricts the amount of exercise you should do, consult your health care practitioner first.

   Exercise often lowers blood cholesterol in your body and may decrease the severity of atherosclerosis (buildup of fatty deposits in the arteries). Such exercises as jogging, swimming, walking, and bicycling are most effective. (See the section on exercise in Chapter 2.)

TREATMENT:

There is no cure for high blood pressure; however, it can be controlled after prompt diagnosis through diet; modification of life style; and medication, if necessary.

Since prevention and treatment of high blood pressure are essentially the same, the measures listed above under "Prevention" are applicable to treatment as well. That is, you should stop smoking; lose weight if necessary; decrease the amount of sodium/salt, cholesterol, and saturated fat in your diet; reduce stress; and exercise regularly. In mild high blood pressure, this may be all the treatment that is needed. In other cases, however, medication to lower blood pressure may be necessary in addition to these measures.

There are several major categories of medication to control high blood pressure. The most commonly used are diuretics (water pills). Diuretics help the kidneys to get rid of salt as well as water which decrease the blood volume in the body and lower the blood pressure to a desirable level. However, *some* diuretic medications promote loss of potassium, and supplements may need to be taken as prescribed by a health care practitioner. Examples of diuretics: Lasix, Hygroton, Esidrex, Dyrenium, Aldactone, Dyazide.

The second group of medications acts directly on the blood vessels by opening up the narrowed arterioles (small arteries). Example: apresoline (hydralazine).

The third group acts on the nervous system by relaxing the tightened and narrowed arteries and arterioles, thus allowing the blood to flow more easily. Examples: Aldomet, Minipress, Catapres (clonidine).

The fourth group decreases the work of the heart by blocking the body's response to adrenalin, thus lowering blood pressure. Examples: Inderal, Lopressor.

All the medications that are used to control high blood pressure should be taken regularly under the supervision of a health care practitioner.

The thought of taking medication for an extended period of time, possibly for the rest of one's life, may not be particularly appealing. However, we are fortunate that high blood pressure can be controlled through treatment. The benefits of control (decreased risk of heart disease, stroke, increased life expectancy) are too great to ignore.

Medications used to treat high blood pressure can cause side effects. Some of these are minor and may decrease with time; others may be more unpleasant. It is important to be aware of the side effects of the particular medication you are taking so that you may report their occurrence to your health care practitioner. If side effects occur, or if treatment is not successful, your practitioner may try several different medications or combinations of medications to find what works best for you.

It is not wise to skip, stop, or increase your medication unless told to do so by your health professional. If stopped abruptly, some medications may cause serious side effects such as a very rapid rise in blood pressure, an irregular heartbeat, or a heart attack.

Osteoporosis

Osteoporosis is a common bone disease that occurs primarily in women past menopause. It can be defined as a decrease in the overall bone mass present in the body. The bones become thin and brittle, and fractures may occur with little or no cause (spontaneous fractures). The bones most often affected are the weight-bearing ones of the lower spine and hip and bones of the wrist.

CAUSE:

Osteoporosis is apparently caused by a combination of hormonal, nutritional, and physical factors. There is some bone loss in all people as aging progresses. This bone loss accelerates in women at menopause when estrogen levels in the body decrease. (Estrogen seems to have a protective effect on bone.)

Another contributing factor is long-term inadequate intake of calcium. Calcium is necessary for strong bones as well as for proper functioning of nerves, muscles, and cells. Since the calcium level in the blood must remain fairly constant even if there is a low dietary intake, calcium is removed from the bones when necessary to make up the deficit. If this occurs over a long period of time, weaker bone is the result.

Other factors which increase the risk of developing osteoporosis are a family history of osteoporosis, a small body frame, thinness, cigarette smoking, and a sedentary way of life. It is more common among whites than blacks.

Some medications, when taken for long periods of time, may contribute to osteoporosis either by decreasing calcium absorption or by increasing calcium excretion from the body. These include steroids (often used to treat rheumatoid arthritis), heparin, aluminum-containing antacids, and the diuretic furosemide (Lasix).

WHY WOMEN?:

Osteoporosis occurs in approximately one in four postmenopausal white women in the United States. Although it does occur in men, women are more likely to develop osteoporosis for a variety of reasons. Women tend to have less bone mass than do men. They also live longer than men do. Women are most likely to go on reducing diets throughout their lifetimes: when weight is lost, so is bone. If a woman does not maintain an adequate calcium intake during pregnancy and breast feeding, her calcium stores are used by the baby. Also, many women erroneously believe that adults do not need milk. This results in a chronic shortage of calcium in the diet.

SYMPTOMS:

Unfortunately, there may be no symptoms for many years after the disease process has begun. Often a bone fracture is the first indication that osteoporosis is present. Osteoporosis is often first seen on an x-ray which was performed for another reason.

Signs and symptoms which may occur include progressive loss of height over the years, "dowager's hump," and low back pain or back muscle spasm.

An interesting theory proposed by researchers is that periodontal disease may be an early sign of os-

teoporosis, occurring five to ten years before osteoporosis is noted in the rest of the body.

PREVENTION:
   Prevention is the best treatment for osteoporosis
and is concentrated in two areas: regular exercise
and adequate calcium intake.

TREATMENT:
   The goals of treatment are to maintain the bone
which remains and to prevent additional loss. If osteoporosis is severe, nothing will restore the affected
bone to normalcy.
   Treatment consists of regular exercise, adequate
calcium intake, and possibly estrogen therapy.
Treatment with estrogen is controversial because it
increases the risk of developing endometrial cancer
(cancer of the lining of the uterus) as well as gall
bladder disease and heart disease. Unlike treatment
for postmenopausal symptoms, estrogen therapy for
osteoporosis may continue for many years. This is
an important consideration because the risk of endometrial cancer is both time- and dose-related.
This means that the risk is greater the higher dosage
and the longer the treatment lasts. (See the section
on cancer earlier in this chapter.)
   Estrogen therapy may be given as a preventive
measure to women thought to be at a particularly
high risk to develop osteoporosis.
   The search for a safer and more effective treatment than estrogen therapy is under way. Some researchers are studying combinations of drugs, such
as calcium, estrogen, and sodium fluoride; others

are studying the effects of some forms of vitamin D. However, all these treatments are still in the experimental stage.

Senility

"Senility" is a frightening word. Both to the general public and to many health professionals, it implies severe, irreversible mental deterioration, dependence, and loss of bodily control. Many people think that it is an inevitable part of aging. These misconceptions help perpetuate the myth that senility is a single entity without a cure.

Senility is *not* a normal part of aging. In fact, "senility" is a rather vague term used to describe a great number of conditions, of which many are curable and others can be improved. The corresponding medical term "senile dementia" is equally vague. Recently, an attempt has been made by the health professions to define "dementia" more precisely and to differentiate it from other illnesses in which confusion or memory loss may be symptoms.

Dementia is a deterioration in mental function which usually occurs gradually over a period of time and which may involve intelligence, mood, memory, judgment, and orientation. Approximately 10 to 20 percent of people over age 65 have significant mental impairment. Of these, up to 40 percent have potentially curable or treatable conditions.

It is important to remember that occasional forgetfulness is normal at any age. Symptoms such as confusion, memory loss, personality changes, and inability to concentrate do not necessarily indicate dementia. They may be caused by medications; depression; thyroid problems; vitamin B_{12} deficiency; heart, lung, kidney, or liver disease; tumors; high fever; head injury; and alcoholism. When these conditions are treated, the dementialike symptoms decrease or disappear completely. It is a great tragedy that many older people are misdiagnosed as senile when they are actually suffering from a curable illness or condition. That is why it is important that anyone with such symptoms have thorough physical, neurological, and psychiatric examinations which include a detailed medical and personal history to attempt to determine their cause. If the individual cannot provide such a comprehensive history, then a knowledgeable relative or friend should be consulted.

Even if the illness is not curable, much can be done to reduce symptoms and to help both the individual and her family to better cope with them.

The two main causes of incurable dementia are Alzheimer's disease (60 percent) and multi-infarct dementia (20 percent). In Alzheimer's disease changes in the brain's nerve cells prevent them from working properly, thereby decreasing the number of functioning brain cells. It occurs more often in women than in men and can occur in middle age as well as in older people. The cause of Alzheimer's disease is unknown.

In multi-infarct dementia, blood clots block many of the small arteries throughout the brain, causing destruction of brain cells. High blood pres-

sure and possibly diabetes are thought to be underlying causes.

Treatment for dementia revolves around reducing symptoms when possible, establishing ways to
deal with symptoms which do not respond to treatment, and individual and family counseling to help
those involved to better cope. The goal of treatment
is to maintain and/or to improve functional ability.
General health measures such as proper rest, a nutritious diet, regular exercise, and good personal hygiene are recommended. It is important to maintain
daily routines, social contacts, and intellectual stimulation. Memory aids such as a calendar; a written
activities list; labels on household items; and verbal
reminders of time, place, and person help people
help themselves. On rare occasions medication may
be used to treat depression, agitation, or insomnia.
(In general, medication use in dementia is severely
limited because of potentially serious side effects.)

Both individuals and their families can benefit
from group and individual counseling. Increased
publicity about these illnesses and their problems in
recent years has led to the establishment of family
support groups across the country. In addition, researchers continue to look for the causes of dementia as well as for an effective treatment. Studies
using choline, procaine, hormones, and other medications to treat dementia have been inconclusive so
far.

Although little is known about prevention of dementia, it is considered important to maintain op-
timum mental functioning. Older people should

stay mentally and physically active and develop outside interests, hobbies, and other activities. Adequate rest, regular exercise, and a balanced diet are also recommended. It is important to tend to minor illnesses immediately and to avoid unnecessary medications. Early detection and treatment of high blood pressure will help prevent multi-infarct dementia.

Urinary and Gynecological Problems

URINARY TRACT INFECTION:

The possibility of developing a urinary tract infection increases rapidly after age 65. This is apparently the result of changes in the aging bladder which increase its susceptibility to infection. For example, the muscle tone of the bladder decreases, so that it may not empty completely. Hormonal changes after menopause (decreased estrogen levels) also increase the likelihood of developing an infection, as do inactivity and a poor nutritional state. Diabetics are at higher risk.

Symptoms of a urinary tract infection include pain or burning on urination, frequent urination, a feeling of urgency to urinate, incontinence (inability to control the urge to urinate), and pain and fullness in the lower abdomen.

Diagnosis is usually made by urinalysis, and by urine culture, if necessary. If the urinalysis shows the presence of pus and bacteria, the urine is cultured to identify the bacteria. The bacteria are then tested for their sensitivity to different antibiotics.

Treatment is instituted with the antibiotic found to be most effective and is continued for one to two weeks. A repeat culture should be performed to make sure that the infection has been cured.

Other measures recommended to treat urinary tract infection and to prevent its recurrence are:

1. Increase fluid intake, especially water. Cranberry juice may be recommended to make the urine more acidic.
2. Take showers instead of baths.
3. Avoid bubble baths, perfumed soaps, and feminine hygiene sprays.
4. Wear cotton panties.
5. Avoid harsh laundry soaps and bleaches and rinse clothes well.
6. Avoid pantyhose next to the body and tight slacks.
7. Wipe from front to back with a single stroke when toileting.
8. When on a long car trip, stop every few hours to urinate.
9. Cleanse the anal area thoroughly after each bowel movement.

STRESS INCONTINENCE:

Stress incontinence occurs when urine is lost involuntarily while coughing or straining. It is usually caused by loss of tone in the muscles which support the bladder, vagina, and rectum, but it may also occur because of urinary tract or vaginal infection or urinary obstruction. If the incontinence is caused by infection, treatment with the appropriate anti-biotics should cure it.

To treat (and prevent) stress incontinence caused by weak pelvic muscles (the most common cause), the muscles can be strengthened by daily practice of Kegel's exercises, also called pelvic floor exercises.

To do these exercises, concentrate on alternately relaxing and contracting the muscles you use to stop and start urination, the vaginal muscles, and the rectal muscles you use to stop and start bowel movement. Slowly contract and relax these muscles five or six times and gradually work up to doing this several times a day. You can also practice this when urinating. You are using the correct muscles if you can start and then stop the flow of urine several times during urination.

Here are some other preventive measures:

1. Try to urinate every three hours or so.
2. Avoid severe constipation, which can cause incontinence by fecal impaction.
3. Limit fluids at bedtime; be sure to drink enough fluid during the day, however.
4. Limit alcohol and tea, coffee, or other caffeine-containing beverages.

In some instances the muscles can be surgically repaired.

VAGINITIS:
Most gynecological problems which develop among older women occur because estrogen levels

in the body are greatly decreased after menopause. With decreased estrogen levels, the walls of the vagina become smooth, thin, and dry and are easily irritated. The acidity of the vagina also decreases, creating favorable conditions for growth of bacteria. Irritation or infection of the vagina (atrophic or senile vaginitis) are the most common gynecological complaints among older women. The usual symptoms are itching, a pink-tinged discharge, and pain during intercourse. Sometimes urinary symptoms such as frequent urination or pain or burning on urination occur.

If pain with intercourse is the only symptom, the use of a water-soluble lubricant such as K–Y Jelly is recommended during intercourse. Continued sexual activity helps counteract vaginal dryness. If other symptoms are present, the usual treatment is the application of a vaginal estrogen cream. The cream is used nightly at first; the dose is eventually reduced to twice a week. If an infection is also present, an antibiotic cream is also prescribed.

The cream is considered a safe alternative to oral estrogen therapy, which may increase the risk of developing cancer of the lining of the uterus. However, some estrogen is absorbed into the body when the cream is used, and the long-term consequences of this have not been established.

VAGINAL BLEEDING:

It is not normal to have any vaginal bleeding after menopause. Bleeding may occur for many reasons. It may be caused by vaginitis, cervical polyps, oral estrogen therapy, or cancer of the uterus or ovaries. Therefore, if bleeding does occur, it is important to have it evaluated by your health care practitioner as soon as possible.

SUGGESTIONS FOR MAINTAINING
GYNECOLOGICAL HEALTH:

A pelvic examination, including a speculum examination, is recommended once a year. A pap smear is usually necessary only once every two to three years. If the regular-size speculum is uncomfortable, ask that a smaller speculum be used. Since many women find it difficult to talk about gynecological problems and embarrassing to have them, search for an understanding health care practitioner with whom you feel comfortable.

Weight Control

Millions of Americans are overweight, including unfortunately, a substantial percentage of older women. In addition, a large number of women over 50 are obese, that is, 20 percent over desirable weight. Desirable weight or ideal body weight (IBW) is determined by age, sex, height, body build, and ideally by the proportion of muscle and fat in the body. A good barometer of what we should weigh now is our weight at age 25, as long as that was within a normal range.

We have a tendency to gain weight as we get older because although we are usually less active, and therefore burning fewer calories, we continue to eat as much or more than we did in our twenties. Also, as we age our metabolism slows down (using less calories), and a higher percentage of our bodies is fat (fat is a more efficient user of calories than is muscle). Physiologically, women have a higher percentage of body fat than men do. This is nature's way of protecting the growing baby during pregnancy and breast feeding. This extra fat often makes it harder for women to lose weight.

Some people are plagued with particularly efficient metabolic systems which make maximum use of calories consumed. This is a throwback to an earlier stage of existence when survival depended on body storage of extra calories for lean times.

Psychologically, this is a thin society in which those who are overweight or obese may be stigmatized as unattractive or lacking in willpower and self-control. We come in all shapes and sizes and some of us will never be skinny, nor should we want to be. How we feel about ourselves and our weight should not be determined by society's unrealistic expectations.

There are health reasons why none of us should be obese, however. Obesity is considered a risk factor for heart disease, atherosclerosis, high blood pressure, diabetes, and gall bladder disease; and it may make surgery difficult or more dangerous. Weight loss is part of the treatment for high blood pressure, heart disease, diabetes, and arthritis. Extra weight puts great strain on the back, hips, and knees, making arthritis more painful and harder to control. Losing weight can lower the blood pressure, decrease the need for medication, and help control blood sugar in diabetes.

If you decide that it would be best for you to lose some weight, your first step should be to discuss your plans with your health care practitioner. You both should decide on a weight-loss goal and how you plan to reach it. Weight loss should be gradual—one to two pounds per week. Very stringent reducing diets or very rapid weight loss can be particularly dangerous for older people. Your health care practitioner should be able to provide you with sample meal plans and calorie charts. The best way to lose weight is to cut down on the amount of food you eat, especially by cutting out high-calorie, low-nutrition foods, while increasing your activity.

HERE ARE SOME OTHER HINTS:
1. Plan nutritionally balanced meals using foods from the four basic food groups every day. (See the section on nutrition in Chapter 2.) By doing this you are cutting just calories, not nutrients. Nutritionally adequate, satisfying meals will maintain your good health while helping you stay on your reducing diet and reeducating your eating habits.
2. Think of weight loss as a challenge, not as a chore. You will be more successful if you plan your reducing diet around the foods you like, but cut down on portion size, change the method of preparation, and/or substitute low-calorie alternatives. For example: steam, poach, or broil instead of frying or sautéing;

substitute skim milk for whole milk; substitute low-fat yogurt for sour cream; eat fruit for dessert or cut portions of high-calorie sweets in half.

3. Increase your daily activity. Studies have shown that many overweight people actually eat less than their thin peers but are much more sedentary. It is very difficult to lose weight only by reducing calories. Therefore, if you can, walk instead of taking the bus, use stairs instead of elevators, and plan an outdoor activity to get you moving each day.

4. Begin a regular exercise program. Exercise has a dual benefit, since it speeds up metabolism (using up calories) while it suppresses the appetite. Suggested exercises are walking, jogging, swimming, or cycling. (See the section on exercise in Chapter 2.)

5. Do you eat to reward yourself? When you are not hungry? To be polite? When you are anxious? To lose weight and to maintain that loss it is necessary to stop those unhealthy eating habits and to adopt healthy ones. Some people, by recognizing in what circumstances they overeat, are able to change such behavior patterns on their own. However, many people need the support and guidance of others. Groups such as Weight Watchers and Overeaters Anonymous offer such assistance. In any case, it is almost impossible to maintain a permanent weight loss unless faulty eating patterns are corrected.

a) Don't food-shop when hungry. Use a grocery list and plan your food budget and stick to it. That way you will save money as well as calories.

b) Do not keep high-calorie snacks such as candy, cookies, and baked goods around to tempt you. Instead, stock fresh or dried fruit and vegetables, and fruit juices.

c) Food should not be used as a reward. Treat yourself to a movie, a paperback book, a pretty scarf, or a bubble bath instead. These contain no calories and they last longer.

d) Eat slowly and concentrate on what you are eating. Overeaters often eat very quickly and do not realize how much they consume. Do not watch television or read while eating.

e) Eat breakfast. A good breakfast provides energy and nutrients to start the day, helps you to avoid high-calorie mid-morning snacks, and prevents you from overeating at lunch. Studies have shown that many overweight people skip breakfast and/or lunch only to gorge themselves at dinner and bedtime.

6. Every few months a new reducing diet appears on the scene offering quick weight loss with little effort. Recently these have included the high protein, low-carbohydrate, diet (Stillman, Atkins, Scarsdale), high-carbohy-

drate, low-protein diet (another Stillman), the egg and grapefruit diet, the "all-you-can-eat" diet, and so on. Basically, all these diets are variations of the standard low-calorie reducing diet, but none is nutritionally balanced. Some are high in fat and cholesterol; some are deficient in protein and vitamins. There may be rapid initial weight loss, mainly from water loss, but this is not a permanent loss. These diets do not work in the long run because they are impossible to maintain over a long period of time, are not nutritionally adequate, and do not permanently change eating habits. Therefore, weight is regained after the diet is stopped. None of the fad diets provides the permanent weight loss which is the goal of dieters. Many overweight Americans try each fad diet as it appears, losing nothing in the long run but their hard-earned money. Unfortunately, there is no easy, effortless way to lose weight. It takes motivation, discipline, and concentration. Calories *do* count.

7. "Diet pills," such as over-the-counter appetite suppressants, may help you lose weight temporarily, but weight is usually regained after they are stopped, since they do not change eating habits. These drugs usually contain caffeine, which may cause jitteriness, nervousness, insomnia, and heart palpitations and are not recommended as weight-loss aids. Other medications such as hor-

mones or amphetamines are dangerous drugs with serious side effects and should never be used to lose weight.

8. Weigh yourself once a week. With gradual weight loss you will usually not see a difference every day.

9. It is all right to have a high-calorie dessert or snack occasionally; but be especially careful of what you eat the next day. Extra pounds mount up quickly. It is easier to lose five pounds than twenty-five pounds.

10. Do not get discouraged. Losing weight is hard work and takes both time and patience.

FIVE

Social Relationships

No life is isolated. From the minute we are born until the minute we die, we stand in relation to others—to the small world of our families, to the larger one of our community, to the world. Throughout our lives, we play different roles within these circles of relationships. We are born daughters; we become mothers. We are born dependent; we become caregivers.

The focus here is the problem of changing relationships caused by aging. But the real issue is not how we relate to children, grandchildren, husbands, lovers, and friends but how each of us can take control over our individual lives and direct their course until they are completed.

We have presumed to make some suggestions, but we are very aware that the real solutions will come from within, from the courage and wisdom amassed through living.

For a long time the Western world has tended to look at life as if it were a tidy hill. Supposedly, we climb up the hill as we mature, stand briefly on the top, then begin the long, slow walk down and out of the picture. One side of the hill is supposed to be matched point for point on the other side—adolescence is matched with mid-life crisis, babyhood with senility, birth with death. The seven ages of man, taken from Shakespeare's *As You Like It,* glorifies this concept. The ageism inherent in society makes us believe that it is real, that after a certain point, the longer we live, the more powerless we become.

But the hill does not exist. It is a myth. Our lives are not neat bell-shaped curves; there are adventures that contribute to human history from beginning to end. When we really understand this, the idea of a rising and declining life will have no power over us. Even if the ageists in our society still believe in it. Many people after Galileo still believed that the sun revolved around the earth, but once the truth was known, they could be laughed at as slightly nutty crackpots. Any false idea loses the ability to hurt once enough people begin to see its falseness. Maggie Kuhn writes:

If we could stimulate a life review, we would see what we have lived through, the ways in which we have coped and survived, the changes we have seen—all of this is the history of the race. Older Americans have lived through more changes than any other human group. If we do not see the value of this experience because of our society's foolishness and our lack of insight as to what makes human beings really human, we will have done great damage to ourselves and to those who come after. . . . I feel that old people have a particular responsibility in our society to develop, test, and try on for size some new roles. The roles are patterned after the model of the elders of the tribe, who are responsible for the tribe's survival and those who come after. There is absolutely no excuse for any of us to retreat to our own private worlds because of our age.

SOCIAL ROLES

Caregiving

From our very youngest years, we learned that one of our basic roles in life is that of caregiver. First we mothered our dolls, fed them from tiny dishes, dressed them, bandaged them, sewed clothes for them. Later, we took care of our younger brothers and sisters, helped with dinner and the dishes, and worked around the house. Our first paid job was probably watching a neighbor's children. If we trained for work, we most often trained for a caregiving occupation—nurse, teacher, secretary. It has become second nature for us to remember the favorite foods of those close to us, to soothe scraped knees and plan birthday parties, to be there when someone needs us, to think of another person's well-being before our own.

This socialization can cause many problems for women. As daughters, wives, mothers, and friends, we learn that we are expected to give. It is assumed that we will always provide care for others even if it means not taking care of ourselves. Hospital social workers and staff automatically conclude that if there is a daughter or daughter-in-law she will provide home care for the chronically sick older parent in a family. In fact, family supports, provided mainly by women, are responsible for 80 percent of all human services given to the older, chronically ill person.

Furthermore, encouraged by the woman's movement in the late 1960s and the 1970s, and prompted by the steady rise of the cost of living, many women joined the work force in middle age. Forty-two percent of all women between the ages of 55 and 64 are employed outside the home. And often the income from that work has become a family necessity.

As a result, the 60-year-old woman may be caring for an 80-year-old parent or in-law as well as holding down a full-time job. This woman, described by Elaine Brody, prominent gerontologist, as the "woman in the middle," may also find that her grown children are returning home because of divorce or economic hardship. Very often grandchildren will be added to the list of those who need her care.

"Home is where you go and they have to take you in," wrote the poet Robert Frost. But sometimes family counseling may be necessary to help children become less dependent or to help an overburdened mother to learn to say no. It is important that the rewards of continuing care for children and their children are not offset by the problems.

The decisions that have to be made about whether to provide home care for an older person who is not able to care for himself or herself are often difficult ones. Great conflict can arise in a family faced with the additional needs of an older relative. As many plans as possible should be made before there is a crisis. It is difficult to plan carefully or consider alternatives during critical times. The person who will need care deserves to participate in these discussions. The person who will be responsible for the major portion of that care should be supported and urged to speak honestly, to assess the reality of the situation, and to recognize limitations and feelings.

If you are considering taking care of an older relative, you might think about some or all of the following.

It is not necessarily a solution to say that you should give up work. It is often difficult to sacrifice your income, job satisfaction, and independence to be at home. These sacrifices cause stress, often felt by the whole family, and create more problems than they solve. Another approach may have to be tried.

It is understandable to resent the needs of the person who requires care. At times you will be overcome with fatigue and anxiety. You will often feel that there is no time for yourself. It is also painful to watch someone you love become sicker and more dependent, to watch a formerly strong person become less and less able. It can be threatening, making you fear the time when you may need help. Older women, especially those in caregiving roles, have told us that they worry a lot about "becoming a burden" on their families later.

Make sure that you know what community supports are available to allow you to have time for yourself. If the family can afford it, you can hire assistance through private agencies that ranges from shopping and housekeeping to personal health assistance. Government agencies, through Medicaid, can provide some help to the homebound if he or she is deemed indigent, although this help is scarcely adequate. There is pending legislation to expand services and to provide tax credits to families to offset the costs of private help. Medicare provides limited support for home care.

Find a support group for caregivers. These groups provide emotional support as well as practical information about available health services and legislative issues. Sometimes these groups are able to offer the services of an attendant to provide respite care while you come to meetings.

Insist on sharing responsibility. Get a commitment for relief hours from your family. If you resist help and forego your own needs for sleep, nutrition, and social activities, you will be in real danger of becoming sick yourself.

Even if you are not concerned about your own health and emotional well-being and are willing to sacrifice yourself to care for a family member, realize that the stronger you are, the better care you can provide, that the hours you spend away give you rest, so that you will come back to your work with new energy.

CAREGIVING IN MARRIAGE:

Marriage is never easy, and chronic illness can increase existing tensions and add new ones. Often, economic strain, lessening of sexual desire and activity, and a decrease of shared interests and activities combine with resentment and anger. In a good marriage, partners nurture each other. When one partner needs care for a long time, the other must increase the amount of nurturing, often getting nothing in return, not even thanks.

Because in general women live longer than men and usually marry persons older than they are, they often become caretakers for their chronically ill husbands later in life.

Most women want to spare their husbands nursing home placement "at all costs," and by doing this they take work upon themselves that is physically and emotionally draining. Taking care of an invalid, especially a person who is frail and/or bedridden and gets steadily worse, is hard work. The woman who slept "with one ear open" to listen for a baby crying in the night or a teenager coming home from a party now listens for her husband's requests for help.

One woman confided. "Sometimes he can't make it to the bathroom in time, and then I have to get up to change the sheets; sometimes he's so afraid he says, 'Sit with me. Just hold my hand.' I'll sit there for hours. When I try to go back to bed he wakes up, begs me to stay. I'm so tired, I want to die just so I can sleep."

In addition, the wife's continual lifting and supporting, along with doing the laundry, the cleaning, and the shopping and cooking for a finicky appetite on a special diet, as well as driving to health professionals' appointments, when combined with inadequate rest and her own aging can lead to a pain-filled, sleep-walking existence.

Not only must this woman frequently do the work of a stevedore, but she must bear terrible emotional burdens as well. She must watch someone she loves and has depended on deteriorate bit by bit. That he might die at any time is a constant fear, and contemplating his death will often force her to have to contemplate her own. The man who has always been the producer, has always been active, will often resent his condition and take out his resentment on the wife who cares for him. Some people express fear as anger, and some illnesses or medications can cause a person to behave violently.

Until recently, care of the dying has not been treated as a special kind of caregiving. But now more and more attention is being given to the needs of those who are completing their lives. The following are suggestions for those who care for the dying.

It is important to realize that the person who is dying is first a person and that dying is part of his or her life. Most of us are afraid of death and afraid to think about it. When the dying person wants to talk about the future, our first reaction may be to change the subject or to make some hearty and false statements like: "*You're* not dying. You look better every day," or "You'll live longer than any of us."

But dismissing the subject will isolate the dying person and make communication almost impossible even between people who have always been close. Often someone's expressions of grief, fear, anger, and hopelessness are very uncomfortable to be around. But these feelings need to be expressed before people can reconcile themselves to any painful condition and accept it.

Those who care for the dying do not need to worry about how to bring the subject up or what to say when the dying person wants to talk. Cecily Saunders, founder of the hospice movement, reminds us that the real issue is what we let the dying *tell us*. Listening with loving attention as often as we can is the most important thing we can do.

The dying want those around them to be cheerful and pleasant. A caregiver's sense of humor can help both her and the person she is caring for to bear the unbearable, think the unthinkable, and say the unsayable.

The dying fear abandonment. If it is possible, frequent visits from the same people can help to ease these fears. Because of this, family members should put aside old battles and work together to support the dying member and each other.

Children are the future and one form of immortality. Their visits are special. They should be encouraged, but not forced, to visit.

In selecting a health care practitioner, the patient and caregiver should choose the most competent person available. Competence gives the dying person a sense of security that everything possible is being done in the best way possible. The patient and the caregiver should be able to discuss all aspects of treatment with the health care practitioner as well as the best ways of maintaining both a pain-free and alert life.

When someone is dying, friends don't come around as often as they used to. Some don't come around at all. Worse yet, grown children, frightened by the situation, avoid their parents. The already isolated woman faces losing touch with both children and grandchildren at a time when she desperately needs someone to talk to and to give love that can be returned.

Any illness is expensive. A long-term illness can eat huge holes in a family budget, even when a couple has good medical coverage. Savings are often used up in covering medical costs not taken care of by insurance, and money is then not available to pay for respite care to provide relief for the wife.

Medicare covers all people eligible for Social Security but not adequately.

Home health care and nursing home care are often funded through Medicaid, which provides health care only for the indigent, and so a couple must spend down assets in order to be eligible. This disposing of assets will often leave the wife with very little support during the illness and after the death of her husband.

If you are a caregiving wife, there are some things you can do to help yourself.

1. No matter what you have to do to manage it, find a support group for caregivers and go to meetings. If this is all you can do, do this one thing. You will find out that you are not alone; you will have a place where it is acceptable to

express your sorrow, anger, and resentment. You may also get some practical help and find ways to advocate for change in home care legislation.

2. Your husband may feel sorry for himself or be angry about your need to get away, but your own health can be seriously jeopardized unless you get some relief. You need time away from home. If money is a real problem, perhaps your children can relieve you either by sponsoring some hours of professional home care or by giving some themselves. Your church may also be able to give you some volunteer help. Some women who have large homes are able to trade lodging for respite care with a student or a working person.

3. Find ways to take care of yourself. This situation is life threatening for many women. Take time to eat nutritious meals. Rest when you can. See your health care practitioner when you need to. Avoid alcohol and use tranquilizers sparingly, if at all. Look for other, nonaddictive ways to relieve stress.

4. If your husband is able, work on opening lines of communication. Most people hate their angry, powerless, self-pitying feelings, but they need to express them. If you can listen to his feelings and find a way to express your own, your marriage will grow as a result.

5. Keep in touch with friends and family by letter and telephone. Fight off isolation as much as possible.

6. Finally, remind yourself over and over that you are doing the best, most loving job you can.

If, after all, nursing home placement becomes an option you must consider, do not try to make the decision alone. Although guilt feelings are normal in this situation, there is nothing to feel guilty about. You have not failed. Discuss the situation with your husband's health care practitioner and with your own, and if you can, with your husband and family. If you need more help, find counseling.

Sexuality

Our society has always had trouble accepting sexuality among its older members, particularly older women. Even though more and more studies show that sexual desires are normal throughout life, there is little evidence that this information has been absorbed by the general population. Since we are members of the society, we share its attitudes. After feeling for most of our lives that sexuality in older people is abnormal, as we grow older we begin to have those same feelings about ourselves.

We do not want to belong to a group that is discriminated against, that is "not like everybody else." That is one reason why cosmetic companies and advertising agencies make hundreds of millions of dollars selling products that are supposed to make us look younger. It is why we consider complimentary remarks like, "You certainly don't look (act) 65 (or 50, 70, or 80, etc.). I thought you were younger." It is why we view our aging bodies with feelings ranging from resignation to dread.

The fact that we have female bodies has shaped our lives in hundreds of ways that we are aware of and in many that remain subconscious. And much of our sexuality is tied up with how we feel about those bodies. Sometimes we are tempted to give up on sex because of the negative images we have of our physical selves as we grow older. We respect our bodies less, and we doubt our attractiveness and worth because we are the victims of the ageism prejudice.

We cannot change the attitudes of a whole country without changing our own first. We must give up feeling the powerlessness of the victim. First we need to remind ourselves over and over that the idea of beauty is arbitrary. In the Middle Ages, small breasts and large abdomens were considered beautiful. Rubens's paintings of women are an example of another standard. In China, women with tiny, deformed feet once set the standard for beauty. The standards for beauty in this culture are largely the products of makeup, lighting, and camera angles and are shaped by the fact that, on the average, we spend twenty-six hours a week or more watching advertising-supported magazines which tell us that only the young are beautiful and that only the beautiful are able to enjoy life. (Most advertising is designed to make even younger women feel ugly and uncomfortable.)

We need to reject this false standard of beauty

outright and give our bodies the respect they deserve. Exercise, a nutritious diet, good posture, cleanliness, and rest can make us more attractive, not because they make us younger, but because they make us feel and look like people who relish life. Another thing we can remember is that the people we most like to have around ourselves are not those who are stunningly beautiful but the ones with "glad-to-see-you" smiles and interested eyes. We can rephrase those so-called compliments by telling people, "No, I don't look younger. This is how a person my age looks and acts."

There are numbers of us who live happy, satisfied, well-adjusted lives who have elected to live them without sex, and there are many more of us who are comfortable with abstinence and willingly choose it at menopause or because of illness or after the death of a loved partner. This is a valid choice. And the people who make it deserve support. Sex is a pleasure and a joy, but it is not essential to a good life.

On the other hand, for those of us who enjoy it, who find pleasure and fulfillment in physical intimacy, sex can be a celebration of our bodies and our womanhood throughout life. Robert Butler and Myrna Lewis write in *Sex After Sixty:*

Sexuality, the physical and emotional responsiveness to sexual stimuli, goes beyond the sex urge and the sex act. For many older people it offers the opportunity to express not only passion but affection, esteem and loyalty. It provides affirmative evidence that one can count on one's body and its functioning. It allows people to assert themselves positively. It carries with it the possibility of excitement and romance. It expresses delight in being alive. It offers a continuous challenge to grow and change in new directions.

NORMAL SEXUAL CHANGE IN AGING:

There is almost no change in a woman's capacity to have intercourse as she grows older. However, vaginal lubrication may take from one to three minutes longer than for a younger woman. Gradually, the lining of the vagina begins to thin and shorten. This may cause some irritation and discomfort during intercourse. The bladder and urethra are less protected and may also become irritated.

Check with your health care practitioner to make sure that any discomfort you have is the result of normal aging. She or he should make it possible for you to be frank about any complaints you have. If your problems are being taken lightly or patronizingly, point this out. Remember, this woman or man may also have some ageist attitudes. You have a right to your sexuality, and if you still are not taken seriously, you may want to find another health professional to consult.

A LITTLE ABOUT MEN:

Normal aging does not usually interfere with a man's ability to have sexual relations. Generally, however, it takes a man longer to achieve an erection and reach a climax, and there is a greater length of time between erections.

Performance fears and anxiety are often causes of impotence in men. Undemanding, considerate, relaxed lovemaking can help the man who worries about losing his masculinity.

Sometimes physical problems can cause impotence. A health care practitioner can check on this possibility. But try to suggest an office visit with all the tact you possess. Often, demands that a man "do something, see somebody" can make psychological aspects of the problem worse.

SOME PROBLEMS:

Lack of partners. There are more older women than older men. In addition, it is more acceptable, even traditional, for men to seek partners among younger women. You might often have to initiate relationships and to consider looking for partners among younger men, which can mean having to break the patterns of a lifetime.

Sex without a partner means masturbation. There is no medical proscription against self-stimulation. In fact, it is often physically very beneficial. However, some people, for social or religious reasons, feel uncomfortable or ashamed about masturbation. Sexual experiences ought to be enjoyable, and the decision about whether to have a particular kind should be one that you make privately. If you feel silly or embarrassed, try masturbating anyway. You might be surprised at how easily those feelings disappear. But guilt and shame are different. The harm they do may outweigh any physical benefits or pleasure the experience will have.

Arthritis. The person with arthritis or osteoporosis may have special problems about self-image, and disability can hamper performance during lovemaking. However, there is some evidence that sex is beneficial for those who have this disease. Experiment with the time of day you make love and with positions. Baths and mild exercise before sex can help you to loosen up and relax.

Heart disease. Consult your health care practitioner if you are not sure about how much exercise is healthy for your heart. She or he can arrange for you to have a stress test if it is necessary. However, sex is usually viewed as a very moderate form of beneficial exercise. If you can walk briskly for three blocks or climb two flights of stairs without shortness of breath, you should have no worries about sexual activity.

Surgery. Surgery is hard on our bodies. Before having any surgery, make sure to ask your surgeon about what to expect afterwards. Ask how it will affect your sexuality and for how long. Insist that you receive answers you can understand. The time it takes for a full medical recovery may be different from the time it takes to feel really good again. If you can, ask other people who have had the same surgery how long it was before they felt "back to normal." You might want to take what they say with a grain of salt, but their answers should give you some sense of how long it is normal to wait before your energy and stamina completely return.

Surgery involving intimate parts of our bodies

can have negative psychological effects on our sexuality. Although hysterectomies, mastectomies, colostomies, and ileostomies need not have physical repercussions on sexuality, counseling may sometimes be necessary for you and/or your partner to work through negative feelings. There are support groups available in many places for women who have had mastectomies and for people who have had colostomies and ileostomies.

Hearing loss. About one quarter of us suffer some hearing loss as we get older. Hearing loss is psychologically disturbing and socially isolating. Because of this, it will have an effect on sexuality and intimacy. If you notice that you miss parts of conversations, or if others notice it and call your attention to it, consult an ear specialist. If your hearing loss can be compensated for with a hearing aid, get one from a reputable dealer and don't let false pride or initial discomfort keep you from using it. For other kinds of deafness there are some surgical procedures which can improve hearing. An ear specialist can advise you. If your hearing loss can't be helped by any of these methods, admit your problem to those around you and ask for help in working out ways to communicate. You may feel awkward, but you will find that others are usually more than willing to give you the help you need.

Drugs. If you notice that your desire for sex has decreased, check with your health care practitioner about the side effects of any drugs you are taking. You should ask about every drug. It is often possible to substitute a drug without this side effect for the one you are taking. Your health care practitioner may also be able to help you figure out how to time your lovemaking so that the drug has the lowest possible effect if a substitution cannot be made or the dosage lowered. However, don't experiment with dosages, substitutions, or times you take a drug without first consulting the person who prescribed it for you.

Alcohol, especially in heavy doses, tranquilizers, caffeine, and the nicotine absorbed in cigarette smoking all have negative effects on the desire for sex.

Privacy. If you live in a nursing home, you may have a hard time finding the privacy you need to engage in sexual activity. Talk about the problem to the administrator in charge of the institution first. If nothing is done, get outside help from your family, friends, clergyman, or lawyer. You might also want to get in touch with advocacy groups such as the Older Woman's League, the Gray Panthers, or the American Association of Retired Persons. A nursing home should not be a prison. Your right to privacy is a basic adult right.

A problem about privacy can also occur if you are living with children or relatives. Talk to your family frankly and insist that ways be worked out for you and your partner to be alone and undisturbed.

There may be times when intercourse is not possible. But sex and sexuality are not expressed only in this way. Intimacy through closeness and touching is also a way of taking pleasure in our bodies and the body of another. These ways of being physically close are almost always available, and they too should be valued as expressions of love and affirmation.

Marriage

In many fairy tales, young lovers must go through all manner of trials and tribulations before they can banish evil and win the right to marry. They can then retire to a blissful "happily ever after" to take care of each other and the new generation of princes and princesses they produce who, in turn, will be the heroes and heroines of a set of new adventures. So the stories go.

The truth is that in the complicated business of living and living together, men and women weave their lives jointly at times, separately at others. Often, men and women become absorbed in their individual lives during middle age, and much of what goes on in a marriage during these years becomes somewhat formalized and automatic.

During these years the woman who worked at homemaking, whose time was spent caring for children, maintaining a house, and establishing a routine centered around that home, has had to face the fact that her children needed her less and less. And as she did so, she felt the sadness and learned about the unexpected pleasures of semiretirement. By the time she is older, she has already coped with the change in her life by establishing different routines and cultivating interests and activities to use the new free times and energy. Often she may have said that she wished she could spend more of this time with her husband.

But when her husband retires from work years later, he may feel bereaved, bored, and restless because he is cut off from the people, places, and work that have absorbed his attention for a long time. Even if a retiring husband has built up serious interests other than those relating to his income-producing work, he will more than likely feel worthless, no longer needed, and often will expect his wife to devote herself full-time to helping him fill the gap left in his life.

Women now complain, good-naturedly for the most part, that their newly retired spouses are nuisances, always underfoot, constantly disrupting their lives.

If both partners retire at roughly the same time, this can place additional stress on individuals who aren't used to being around each other twenty-four hours a day, seven days a week, and if a wife continues to work after her husband has retired, she may find herself and her job the object of her husband's resentment and jealousy. On the other hand, we know a retired husband who delights in his role reversal. He drives his wife to the station, kisses her goodbye, and goes home to work the kinks out of a pâté recipe he's testing. You never know which way the ball will bounce until you try.

At any rate, as you grow older, you and your husband will spend more of your lives together, and it is important to do all you can to make this a joyful, fulfilling time:

1. Find ways to learn to know your husband again and to share yourself with him. You are no longer the same person you were when you married, and neither is he. In the hectic middle years there was little time to really talk or to explore thoughts and reflections. Many couples now take trips and spend time away from the distractions and pressures of home. Even if your income is not large, you can take day trips and, by being in a new environment, begin to grow together and create a new, strong sense of companionship. There will be times of illness and grief ahead, and the closeness you build now will establish a pattern of loving and caring that will be there when it is critically needed. More important, however, is the opportunity it will give you to reap all the joys of a shared life.

2. Do not make abrupt changes in your life style without considering them carefully. Retiring to a community distant from your home may seem like just the thing to alleviate the boredom and restlessness following retirement, but wait until you explore all the possibilities before you move away from the neighborhood or town in which you have lived much of your lives. Even if it is something you have talked about for years, drag your feet for a while and weigh the benefits of a move judiciously against the losses.

3. Use the time you have together to rekindle sexual energies that may have been damped

by too many "too busy, too tired" years. A great deal of our self-worth is invested in the images we have of ourselves as sexual beings. A good sexual relationship can enhance your self-image as well as be enjoyable.

4. Even though it may be especially hard now, keep some part of your life independent and insist that your husband do so, too. If your marriage is still strong after many years, you have probably always done this.

Recognize the legitimacy of your husband's post-retirement distress and allow him to mourn for the part of his life that is now over, but after a time encourage him to develop his own interests and to leave you free to continue yours. A marriage that feeds only on itself will grow weak. Every relationship needs individual contributions to renew and strengthen it. Although you need each other, both of you will feel better about yourselves if you know you can fulfill some of your own needs individually.

Statistically, you will have many healthy years together after retirement. You have always had to work at marriage. Work now to make this a ripe and rich time in your life.

A woman, remembering the last years of her marriage, told us:

We were freer, happier than we had ever been before. We didn't have to worry about our children. We had already done everything for them we could and now they were on their own. My husband didn't have to worry about succeeding at his job. That was over. I did what I liked to do and so did he. And we enjoyed doing things together. Those last years were the best years of our marriage.

Divorce

The mature man usually has a career which provides him with an identity, a means of support, and social contacts outside marriage. Very often, the older woman sacrificed career, education, training, and commitment in order to be a good wife and mother. She and her family have treated her work, if she has done any outside the home, as the dispensable, "help-out" kind, and she has kept her life centered around her husband and family for "better or worse."

While the decision to end a long marriage may be made by a woman who wants to start a new life or may be a mutual recognition that the partners have changed and that a once fulfilling relationship has ceased to grow, most divorces are not the choice of the older woman.

The woman who is told that the marriage to which she has given her life is ending may have some of the feelings created by widowhood and enforced retirement as well as great quantities of rage. And this often happens at a time when her self-image is low, when the media tell her that she is no longer attractive because she is not young. The situation can be especially devastating if the husband is divorcing to remarry. Then society reinforces her feelings of guilt and inadequacy, that she is to blame, that she "couldn't hold her man."

It is important to recognize that the anger and hurt are real. And it is just as important to get appropriate help. Besides individual counseling, self-help and discussion groups are available through community mental health centers, Y's, religious centers, neighborhood centers, or NOW. Sharing the anger, frustration, and loneliness is a good way to begin to cope. Don't wait. Tears are healing and anger creates strength. But feelings of bitterness and helplessness can poison life, and they keep us all from having the freedom we need to grow. Having someone to listen and sympathize is vital at this time, and there is comfort in knowing that you are not the only one to whom this has happened, that others have been there and survived. Group members are also good sources for practical advice.

Avoid, as much as you possibly can, involving children and close family friends. Grown children struggle with as many or more conflicting emotions and loyalties as do younger children of divorcing parents, and they may have fewer ways of getting support. If you can, keep them from taking sides— even yours. It is also important not to cling to your children. You must create a new life for yourself. Going from one dependency to another is not the way to go about it.

Friendships often change as well. Couples who have been friends for years sometimes will find it easier to associate with only one of you. You might also find yourself excluded from some social gatherings because of your new status as a single woman. Friends you valued may need to maintain a distance from both partners until they find new ways to relate to you as individuals. If some friendships are especially important to you and you feel rejected, talk to those couples and tell them how you feel in as direct a way as possible and without asking them to make choices in loyalties. They may be relieved to be able to share their feelings with you, too.

These are some practical issues of particular concern to the older woman going through divorce.

THE LEGAL PROCESS:

1. A good attorney is crucial. An attorney who is a relative or a family friend will have some conflicts no matter how impartial he or she may try to be, so, if at all possible, hire someone who will be able to represent your best interests at all times. The state and local bar associations or women's rights groups can give you names of attorneys to contact.

   Do not share the same attorney with your husband. If there are pressures to do this because "it will be cheaper," the Legal Aid Society can help you to find an attorney of your own. This is one time when you must think of yourself first. No matter how the divorce came about, your life will probably be more difficult than his afterward, and you need to protect yourself in every way you can.

Before hiring an attorney, ask for information about fees and experience with cases such as yours. Talk to others who have employed the attorney in the past. Many good divorce lawyers have worked only with younger couples, and they give their best attention to custody and child support issues. You need someone very experienced in property settlements and support who can advocate for your present and future needs. Methods of splitting property vary greatly from state to state. Even the community-property states (Arizona, California, Idaho, Louisiana, Nevada, New Mexico, Texas, and Washington) do not adhere to the same rules. There is also a debate about what is considered property; in some states property includes pension plans as well as tangible property. Because spousal support, or alimony, can fluctuate with time (usually downward) and the older woman's income can be reduced upon her ex-husband's retirement, your attorney should be very familiar with pension rights, life insurance benefits, Social Security compensation, and health plan coverage.

Seek an initial consultation with the person you want to retain. This will give you a chance to determine whether you are comfortable with this person before you commit yourself to hiring him or her.

2. Lawyers are expensive. Use the time you pay for about advice on legal matters. Avoid the

temptation to use your attorney for emotional support.

3. Find out about your state's laws regarding support and property rights. The more information you have, the more knowledgeable you will be about safeguarding your future.

4. If you have been married close to ten years and can wait, do not file for divorce until the ten-year mark has passed. This will ensure eligibility for your husband's Social Security as a "surviving spouse."

ON GOING TO WORK:

Those of us who matured in the 1930s and 1940s were told that, if we continued our education past high school, we would be better mothers and more knowledgeable wives. If our parents pushed us to learn how to do something, we were frequently reminded that we might not need our skills, might never use them, but they were good to have "just in case something happened."

In most fields the skills women learned "back then" and seldom practiced have become outdated or rusty . New, more complicated certification requirements and licensing procedures have been legislated. In the last ten years, the equipment many of us were trained to use has become obsolete or has been modified until it is almost unrecognizable.

Even if a woman has worked at times during marriage, employers will often recognize only recent work experience as qualifying her to fill a job. And very often older women will find that they are not wanted as employees.

Many women are forced into work that is temporary, hazardous, pays poorly, and is usually without benefits. They fall into the "last hired, first fired" category along with other discriminated-against members of society.

Though the picture is bleak, it is not hopeless.

If there is a junior college, a college, or a university in your area, find out from the women's studies department or department of continuing education what you need to do to be credentialed or brought up to date in the field you have been trained in, or what short-term programs are offered that will lead to employment. These programs are often inexpensive or free. There are also a number of loans and grants that you may be eligible to receive. Women's studies departments usually sponsor counseling and support groups, and most colleges have employment services. If there is no institution of higher education near you, some schools in your area may offer extension division programs, and frequently courses are offered through the high school or the YWCA or YWHA. Also contact the state and federal departments on aging to find out about available employment programs.

If you are under 70 it is illegal for employers to discriminate in hiring you because of your age. Remember this as you look for work. People are paying attention to age discrimination and are beginning to take employers to court.

Avoid commercial training and employment agencies. They are usually expensive and not very helpful. If you are in any doubt about a training course and its usefulness, contact the Better Business Bureau or the consumer rights organization in your area.

FINAL THOUGHTS:

Divorce is never simple or easy. Do all that you can to emphasize your individuality, your power. Do not neglect your health because you are depressed. Find ways to avoid recourse to tranquilizers or alcohol. While you may have to work hard at living for a while, time is usually a great healer.

Remarriage

Marriage is usually thought of as a commitment made by couples during the younger, childbearing years, and our society has traditionally disapproved of marriages that begin in later life. But our life spans have lengthened, and a marriage between older people can bring many years of love, respect, and growth to each partner.

When an older woman's earlier marriage ends with the death of her husband or in divorce, she may choose not to become involved with another man. But if she wishes a woman should feel free to seek a new marriage. Guilt or feelings of disloyalty, of needing to remain "true to his memory," should be looked at, worked through, and gotten over.

There are nearly twice as many older women as there are older men, and this would seem to mean that there are fewer available marriage partners. It is also acceptable for older men to marry younger women, while the converse has been frowned upon. However, there is no evidence anywhere that age difference by itself is a negative factor in establishing a relationship. There are many happy, comfortable marriages with the woman as the older partner.

These are some factors which lead to successful remarriages:

1. Remarriages are happier if both of you know each other well. After many years of living you have developed your own interests, habits, and daily routines. Make sure that these aspects of your lives are compatible. Talk these things over together. Many older people who remarry, marry neighbors or people from the same social circles. Good friendships often grow into more intimate relationships.

2. If possible, move into a new apartment or home. While you both will want to treasure past memories, you are starting a new life together, and a new place to live can be a sign of that life for the two of you. It is also a way of telling children, family, and friends that the two of you are now a couple.

3. Work out all the problems you can with your children and his ahead of time. One of the things they may be concerned about is inheritance rights. This concern may make them feel guilty, and they may not be able to bring the subject up with you. You might be able to avoid a lot of hidden conflict and anger if you can talk to them openly about your plans for

bequeathing any property you have.

Too, even grown children have a hard time accepting a new marriage of an older parent. Many retain the image of parents only as parents linked together in their minds. Remarriage forces them to see you as an independent person choosing a new relationship. It makes you more like they are, and this can be frightening.

However, the decision to remarry is yours. When you discuss this decision with children, discuss it as a decision that has already been made and will not be changed if they disapprove. You are living your life. They will have to accept that just as you have accepted the changes and choices they have made in living their lives.

4. Marriages tend to be more successful when income is sufficient. The financial realities of Social Security are resulting in a growing number of older couples who live together unmarried in order to maintain maximum benefits. This kind of arrangement may not be comfortable for your family, and it may even contradict your own long-held values about how you ought to live. However, as you already know, finances are important in every marriage, and two can only live as cheaply as two. The growth in intimacy with another person does not have to lead to marriage.

5. Finally, if you both have been married before, acknowledge the importance of those relation-

ships in your lives. Marriage is a sharing, and you should be comfortable sharing memories with each other. Work out problems of jealousy, and don't allow comparisons with the past to overwhelm the present relationship and its future.

Widowhood

Widowhood and loneliness are the most overwhelming concerns of older women. The emotional impact of becoming a widow and coping with the loneliness that follows are discussed in Chapter 3, "Mental Health Goals for Older Women." A widow's relations with those around her—children, relatives, and friends—are explored throughout this chapter.

Parenting

The relationships we have throughout our lives with those close to us change as we change. And, while the relationship we have with our children changes too, it is always colored by the fact that at one time we were completely responsible for the very survival of those children, and they were completely dependent on us for that survival.

Much of the growing process involves a striving for independence. "Let *me* do it," children insist almost from the minute they can talk. And, reluctantly at first, we do.

They learn to walk, and after awhile we stop carrying them. They learn to cross streets, ride bicycles, and drive cars. They leave home to go to college, to get jobs, to get married and take on the responsibilities of families of their own. Yet when we look at these tall, strong, competent adults, we also see the helpless babies we once cared for. And when they look at us they see the giants who told them what to do and made everything all right as well as adults growing older, experiencing challenges they cannot yet imagine.

The picture grows even more complicated when we remember that all of us were once children. All of us prize the independence and power that comes with adulthood. It has been hard won. As we become older, one of the things that we most fear is its loss. And our children, as they grow older, want to exercise that power. They want to show us that they know how, that they can do it, do it better than we did. Often, they want to prove their adulthood by trying to direct our lives for us.

For the older woman, this power struggle becomes acute at the times when other transitions are taking place in her life; when she becomes a grandmother or a widow, or at the onset of chronic illness—either hers or her husband's.

Dealing with these conflicts based on emotions that are very old and complicated is not easy. But problems can be solved or ameliorated if we realize that this is a struggle in which the only victory comes through self-awareness and loving compromise.

1. Recognize your children as the adults they

are. Saint Paul said, "When I was a child, I spake as a child. When I became a man, I put away childish things."

Allow them to put away the childish things that embarrass them as they struggle to feel like competent adults. Avoid sentences beginning, "You always were . . ." and "You never did . . ." Every so often try to look at them as people newly met. Write off the little annoyances they make you feel, the way you would for any other person. Take credit for your good parenting and worry about your children when you are alone or with other friends. But when you are with your children allow them to take the credit and responsibility for their own lives. Don't encourage them when they say things like, "I owe it all to you." Doing so would only reinforce an outgrown relationship.

2. Tell them who you are. You are not all-powerful, all-good, or all-wise—and what's more, you never were. It is not a sign of weakness to make such an admission. On the contrary, only a strong person can admit imperfections. By doing this, you are showing your children that you share the imperfections of their own humanity. In some ways this may be painful knowledge. They will want to cling to old images. But they will also want to know these things about you.

One of the hardest things about growing up is realizing that there is no magic, that there is no person you can run to who can fix every-thing. Your children will often come to you with this hope, knowing that they may be dis-appointed. Their disappointment will often take the form of anger. It will help you if you can recognize that this anger is not really an-ger at you but at "the way things are." If you can be matter-of-fact about limitations, you will not only make things easier for yourself but, in the long run, will also help your chil-dren understand that becoming an adult does not mean becoming perfect.

3. Most parents do not want to live with their children, but they would like to live nearby. Often, however, children move away because of their work or marriages, and many parents, on retirement, move to adult communities in more comfortable climates. Sharing the joys and sorrows of each others' lives must then be done through phone calls, letters, and visits.

Visits are certainly the best way for families who don't live near each other to remain close, but they are not perfect. When your children visit you, make sure that there is time for you to enjoy each other alone without in-laws or grandchildren, but it is not necessary to spend every minute together. Also, if at all possible, visit them. Sometimes it is easier for them to come home, but your children will usually en-joy showing you how they live, too.

Once the awkwardness is over and everyone has stopped being on his or her best behavior, look for times to become reacquainted as adults. It goes without saying, of course, that you should avoid giving unsolicited advice about money, housekeeping, marital relations, or child rearing. Instead, remind your children often that you love them and accept the ways they are living their lives. Let them tell you that they love you without brushing it off.

4. Upon becoming widows, many women often notice that the relationships they have with their children begin to change dramatically. They report that grown children act as if their mothers are not capable of making decisions and begin to assume the roles of protectors. Since the death of a husband and father is an emotionally difficult time for everyone, it is usually impossible to act in any planned way or to act according to a set of rules. When your children offer to do things for you, accept their help as you would the help of any good friend. Don't allow them to become responsible for matters that you should control, however. They can come with you to talk to lawyers, bankers, and the like if they are interested, but you must assume the responsibility for your own finances and for everything else that directly concerns you. Do not let them push you into any quick decisions, especially about moving or changing life styles. When they give advice, ask yourself how you would respond if it came from someone outside the family.

Help them with their grief in all the ways you can, but do not let this interfere with your own grieving.

5. If you are facing a debilitating chronic illness, discuss with your children the course of the disease and its implications concerning the care you will require before critical decisions must be made. One good way to do this is to set up a family conference with your health care practitioner and discuss all the possibilities as soon as possible.

Most women have a terrible fear of becoming a burden to their families; at the same time they see nursing home placement as a kind of hell. It is advisable to think about the problems that might be involved in living with your children and to investigate the kinds of health-care-related facilities that are available and to visit them before any decision is made.

You will be able to preserve your independence and take more control over your own life for a longer period if you are able to discuss these matters frankly with your children, as well as plans to be carried out in cases of an emergency or accident.

Grandparenting

Today's grandmothers are very different from the silver-haired stereotypes read about in books and seen on television and in advertising. Statistics reveal that women become grandmothers earlier, often in their forties and early fifties; that many live alone, either divorced or widowed; and that many either work or pursue other activities which take up much of their time and attention.

And families are different. Young families move more often as the primary wage earner becomes more successful. In many cases, a promotion means a move. Grandparents, too, sometimes move to adult communities in other parts of the country after retirement. As a result, many women have to travel great distances to be with their children and grandchildren.

Often there is another complication. The rising divorce and remarriage rate among younger marrieds means that some grandchildren live in families in which neither parent is a relation to the grandmother. Conversely, a woman may find herself the grandmother of children who are not biological descendants.

Stereotypes persist too. Besides the kindly person in the rocking chair, an equally common media picture is that of the meddling whiner (or shrew) who constantly contradicts mothers and fathers and spoils grandchildren rotten (or is too strict). Even though at least one study shows that most activities shared by grandmothers and their grandchildren are initiated by daughters or daughters-in-law or the grandchildren themselves, many women are so frightened of interfering that they carefully limit visits to families.

As a result of all this, 80 percent of today's grandparents see their grandchildren only occasionally.

But children need grandparents. They need the closeness of older adult relatives with whom they can be themselves without worrying about the expectations that come from most normal parents. Grandparents can give their grandchildren confidence, solidity, and a sense of being part of a history. They can make a child feel welcome in the world. "When I was little," a teenager told us, "I loved to be with my gramma. She didn't say much. She never said if she really liked me. But I would have done anything for her."

And grandmothers can derive great benefits from their grandchildren. Relationships with young people are spontaneous and fresh. They are not as colored by the sexism and ageism that comes from long exposure to media images. Young people most often see grandparents as powerful and wise and are fascinated by their interests and perspectives, especially if they are different from those of their parents.

Grandparenting is one of the special benefits of growing older. Following are some suggestions about maintaining contact and developing a relationship with these young people who love and need you.

1. Your grandchildren want to know you. They sense that you have a lot to give them—love, confidence, feelings of roots and family history. If you live close enough, arrange time to visit with them and without their parents. If you are seldom able to see them in person, call just to talk to each grandchild. Ask for him or

her by name and talk only to that person. If you want to talk to your children, call them back later. Remember, too, that mail is almost magical to a child. All those envelopes come every day for other people. Write letters just for a grandchild, sent in envelopes using only his or her name. If you want to send a note to your children at the same time, put it in the envelope with the grandchild's letter. Write to very young children and babies. These letters will become cherished possessions as the child grows older.

If you are close, have your picture taken with your grandchildren and give them a copy. If that is not possible, remember to send them pictures of yourself. They like how you look, and they like being connected with you.

2. You have a right to visit grandchildren whose parents have divorced even if the grandchildren are not living with your daughter or son. If the visits are uncomfortable for you, make them anyway. The special relationship you have with your grandchildren can give them a sense of security and connection with a continuing family which they may badly need.

3. If you are angry or upset with your children or their spouses, tell them, not your grandchildren. This is especially important when a divorce is involved. Do not ask a child to choose sides.

If you feel that your children are talking about you in a negative way around your grandchildren, ask them to stop and to talk over their complaints and criticisms with you. Young people will form a picture of their future relationships with their parents and even their children by the way they see you and your children treat each other.

4. Not all grandparents see less of their grandchildren than they would wish. Divorce, economic pressure, and proximity may create the opposite problem for some grandmothers. Divorced or single-parent daughters and sons often return home with their children, and many expect their mothers to assume full-time care of their children while they work. Many working parents who are reluctant to leave children "with strangers" request full-time baby-sitting help if a grandmother lives close by.

Although you may feel that you have some responsibility to help out in an emergency, you are not obligated to say yes if you are asked to assume full-time care or day care for your grandchildren. You may be delighted to be back in the childrearing business again. But you may not wish to provide care for a second family. Examine your life carefully and make a firm decision that you feel comfortable with.

5. It is normal to have favorites among your grandchildren. They will have favorite grandparents, too. But it is important to offer them all equal opportunity for your time and atten-

tion. As much as you can, be with them one at a time. If they visit you in groups, they will compete for your attention, and you may feel more like a nursery school teacher than a special friend. It goes without saying that gifts should always be equal.

6. Be the kind of grandparent you want to be. If you are the spoiling kind, then spoil. Trust your instincts. Do the things you enjoy most and invite grandchildren to come along. They will probably be delighted. They sense how much you know about how to live.

   On the other hand, some grandparents have a relationship with grandchildren that sociologists call "formal" or "ritual." The grandmother who sends appropriate cards and gifts or is in attendance on special occasions but who has no close, personal friendship with her children's children has a relationship with them which falls into this category. If this describes the kind of contact you have with grandchildren, there is no reason to feel guilty about not being a more "motherly" grandmother. The formal grandmother fills many important needs of her grandchildren.

   Whatever you do, stay in touch with your grandchildren. Margaret Mead wrote:

   In the presence of grandparent and grandchild, past and future merge in the present. . . . Seeing a child as one's grandchild, one can visualize that same child as a grandparent, and with the eyes of another generation one can see other children, just as light-footed and vivid, as eager to learn and know and embrace the world, who must be taken into account—now.

Friendship

Unlike relatives, friends are people with whom we *choose* to spend time and share our lives. Friends provide a kind of support we cannot get from our families.

When we were children, we made good friends with other girls our age. We played together in backyards or on porches; told each other secrets; planned our futures; and formed alliances against the outside world, parents, teachers, and boys. There is something very special about the closeness young girls share.

In junior high school there were gradual changes. We began to compete with each other for attention from boys, and after awhile romantic attachments seemed more important than mere friendships. We started to plan our get-togethers on the nights we didn't have dates. Still, we had a best friend, and when there was a tragedy in our adolescent lives, we talked to her for hours on the phone; spent the night at her house crying, laughing, and eating; and eventually, because she was there, we felt better.

Most of us married and became part of a couple. Managing a home, rearing children, and holding down a job siphoned off energy formerly spent cultivating friendships. Old friends often slid out of our lives as our interests changed or when we moved away, and usually our new friends were, conveniently, partners in compatible couples or mothers of our children's friends.

For those of us who chose not to marry, the attempts to form solid friendships with married women were often frustrating. We seemed to have more hours than our married friends to socialize in the evenings and on weekends, the very times when our married friends most needed and wanted to be with their families. Often, too, we felt uncomfortable in groups primarily made up of couples.

Still, all of us remember friends to whom we could tell things we would never tell anyone else, who shared our lives, who made us comfortable—friends with whom we could be most ourselves.

Our social roles change as we grow older. Often, as we face these changes—children moving far away, retirement, widowhood—we begin to feel that we are useless, that our lives have lost the value they once had. Friends can again make the difference.

The quality of intimacy and support in friendships among older women is often greater than that found among older men or in man-woman friendships. At this stage of life, we have the opportunity and the time to revitalize old friendships and to establish new ones. Sometimes, however, we feel defeated by the loss of those closest to us. We want to shut down our emotions because we feel that we cannot bear any more grief. Another barrier is created when we are willing to accept society's ageist attitudes. "Who would want to be friends with an old lady like me?" we think without examining the truth. The truth is that very few offers of genuine friendship are rejected. There is no life without risk. The support received from friendships, both new and old, will make us healthier persons with more zest for life.

Lesbian Relationships

In this society our value as women is often based on our ability to bear children within a marriage. Tradition holds that women are the keepers of the family and the guardians of a culture based on heterosexual roles.

Large numbers of people in our society view homosexuality as unnatural—a sickness or a sin or both. In many states homosexuals can be jailed. In most states they have no protection against job or housing discrimination. Some have been committed to mental institutions. Many, many more have been cut off from family and close friends.

In literature, movies, and on television, homosexuality is usually presented as a man's "problem." Lesbians, if pictured at all, are often shown as harsh "bad women." Although this is beginning to change, it is still not easy to find portrayals of warm, equal, loving relationships between women.

But many women who married and reared a family because they were afraid of being outcasts feel freer to seek lesbian relationships later in life, even though they face barriers in doing so. Some women who have lived all their lives in small towns or rural settings have had to move to a city to find supporting communities which often provide easier access to lesbian organizations, activities, and places to meet.

But things are beginning to change. At one time bars were often the only places for lesbians to meet each other. But recently organizations have formed to combat discrimination and to provide services and support for lesbian women and gay men. In smaller cities and towns, local women's bookstores often have schedules for socials, consciousness-raising, and discussion groups. Gay and lesbian periodicals will be responsive to the need for information and resources. Often the local NOW chapter will have a lesbian subcommittee.

Two groups for older women are the Gay Older Women's Liberation and the Gay Women's Alternative in New York City. The National Gay Task Force and the Society for Aging and Gay Environment (SAGE) also in New York, can be contacted for information about advocacy issues and about how to get in touch with community groups around the country. Many younger lesbians welcome the addition of older women to the community and take pride in the sense of history they bring with them.

Many older lesbians look forward to retirement as a time when they no longer have to worry about the terrible pressures of hiding their sexual preference in order to keep their jobs. Their lives can become richer and more honest. But the decision to be openly and proudly lesbian takes courage no matter when it is made.

How and when to tell your family and friends is up to you. If you have children, your decision will probably be based on many different considerations. If you live far away from them and don't share much of their lives, it is easier to decide when and if you want to raise the subject. However, if you all live in the same area and see each other often, it may become necessary to talk to them about this important part of your life.

Some children will be supportive, and the trust and respect you have for each other will increase. On the other hand, some will be judgmental and angry. If this is the case, and they are willing, you can work out your feelings together in counseling. There is also group, peer, or one-to-one counseling available for you individually if you need help with anger, guilt, or depression.

But the closeness of a loving relationship is worth seeking. By confronting your fears you can finally find the freedom to live as you choose. Once you decide what you want, there are resources to help you find a community to validate your decision and to give you the support you need to develop and grow.

The broad support of the lesbian community is often crucial for the older lesbian. Having faced so much discrimination during her life, she has good reason to be wary of the formal support system— the doctors, nurses, social and welfare workers—we must all rely on in times of crises. And she is often denied the traditional, informal support given by family and neighbors. The loss of lover(s) and close friends can hurt even more if she has to deny the real nature of her grief. It is extremely important to know who your allies are *before* you have a critical need for them.

There is clearly defined legal discrimination against homosexual couples. It is important for lesbian couples to plan for, and guard against, unequal treatment of each other in cases of the hospitalization or death of one. Make a *legal* will if you have property. Make sure that you and your lover/friend give each other power of attorney in cases of emergency. For husbands and wives, this is automatic, but you will have no rights unless you create them. The National Lawyers Guild or the American Civil Liberties Union (ACLU) can help you find a sympathetic lawyer if you don't know one you trust.

If you can afford it, take out small life insurance policies declaring each other beneficiaries. Doing this can make it possible for your funeral arrangements to be made as you would wish or allow you to make them for your friend/lover.

At times it may seem hopeless when you live in a society that is sexist, ageist, and homophobic. But older women do not have to bear the same isolation as women did in the past. There *are* people to talk to and comfortable ways to develop friendships and support networks.

SIX

Alternative Approaches to Health Care

The medical profession has traditionally been concerned with illness rather than with wellness. It tends to treat the disease, not the person, and thinks about "patients" rather than "consumers" of health care. As we consumers are becoming more aware of ourselves—our bodies, minds, and spirits—we are increasingly dissatisfied with the traditional profession and are turning toward self-help for healthful living and toward alternatives to traditional medicine for alleviation of pain and discomfort.

But a word of caution is needed. Self-help and nontraditional healing as part of the wholistic approach to health are increasingly acceptable to medical professionals and are sometimes recommended by them. However, alternatives to traditional health care should be considered only as a supplement to, never as a *replacement* of, regular care by a health care practitioner. These alternatives should be sought only with the knowledge of a health care practitioner, and after a thorough investigation into the qualifications of the nontraditional practitioner.

This warning applies to all six of the following most generally acceptable nontraditional approaches to health care and healing.

ACUPUNCTURE

Acupuncture is a therapeutic intervention for treating certain painful health conditions. If used with discretion, acupuncture can be helpful to an older person. Well-trained acupuncturists can provide safe relief to people suffering from chronic pain and health problems including arthritis, headaches, overweight, nervousness, allergy, constipation, bursitis, back pain, and sciatica.

The use of acupuncture in the United States is in its infancy in many respects. Although it has been a well-practiced healing technique in China for over five thousand years, its philosophy and effectiveness have not been formally accepted into the legal and medical systems in the United States.

The underlying principles of acupuncture are based on Chinese philosophical approaches to thought and to life in general which view an individual in a wholistic way. This philosophy maintains that the universe is dominated by *ch'i*, a vital life force or energy continually circulating through all living organisms.

Within the human body, *ch'i* flows through specific pathways, or "meridians." According to traditional Chinese approaches to health and disease, when this circulation of *ch'i* is interrupted or blocked in some way, the results will be an imbalance within the body which can cause disease.

The disruption of *ch'i* can be caused by numerous

factors, both internal and external. For example, trauma is considered an externally induced disruption, while emotional pain is an internally caused disruption.

How Is Acupuncture Practiced?

Acupuncture is a technique whereby long, thick needles are passed through the skin to specific points on the body that correspond to the meridians (specific pathways of the flow of *ch'i*). Stimulation of these points is believed to affect and help regulate the flow of *ch'i* to the different organs of the body. The use of acupuncture is not dependent upon drugs, surgery, or hospitalization. At times massage, or acupressure, is utilized as part of the treatment. The treatment is not painful; the needles cause only a slight pinprick sensation.

Acupuncture in America Today

The legal status of acupuncture varies from state to state. The American Medical Association has recognized the use of acupuncture but only as an experimental form of treatment. Many American physicians and medical researchers are studying different theories of acupuncture in an effort to understand how, based on Western scientific principles of medicine and health care, in fact it facilitates healing. Theories studied thus far focus on the involvement of the nervous system, the immune system, as well as the involvement of psychological factors. There is no one explanation of how or why this technique works.

Unfortunately, Medicaid, Medicare, and most private insurance companies do not provide reimbursement for acupuncture practitioners. However, some physicians utilize acupuncture as a component of their regular service, and their service is reimbursable.

As with any health care practitioner, it is important that you find an acupuncturist that you trust and feel comfortable with.

BIOFEEDBACK

Taking responsibility for our own lives and making decisions about the care of our bodies are paramount to maintaining health. The latter involves understanding how our bodies work, learning ways of gaining a greater sense of control over our state of health and well-being, and becoming an active participant in our health care. Biofeedback is one of the most dramatic examples of controlling one's health. Unlike many other techniques discussed in this and other books on health, biofeedback is not a treatment per se but a *learning process* which can help an individual to gain conscious control of her or his body.

The use of biofeedback demonstrates the influence of the mind on the body, and thus the connection between the two. It is a technique involving the use of special instruments to enable a well-motivated person to understand and, to some extent, gain voluntary control over physiological processes that have traditionally been thought to be beyond the realm of conscious control. The autonomic nervous system (ANS) is the principal target of biofeedback training. The ANS is that aspect of the nervous system responsible for the function of glands, smooth muscle tissue, and the heart. Specific functions of the ANS include blood pressure, heart rate, and muscle control.

Biofeedback instruments provide information that can be used to help a person self-regulate certain internal responses. Such instruments have been most effective in monitoring skin temperature, muscle tension, galvanic skin response, and brain waves. The most commonly used biofeedback instrument is the electromyograph (EMG). It monitors a person's muscle activity by giving messages or signals to the subject as visual or auditory cues. The communication is accomplished by placing electrodes on the subject's body.

The use of different types of relaxation techniques is taught to the subject in order to alter the subject's internal responses. Continuous feedback from the machine informs the person of her body's internal state and thus of the progress and the effectiveness of the relaxation technique being practiced. In a sense, the machine acts as a mirror of one's internal physiologic state. Once relaxation is learned, the machine is often no longer needed.

Uses of Biofeedback

The uses of biofeedback include control of migraine headaches, high blood pressure, and cardiac arrythmias (irregular heartbeat); rehabilitation of stroke victims; control of bowel muscles to help regulate incontinence; insomnia; and management of stress.

A specific example is seen in the control of painful migraine headache which is caused by the dilation of the blood vessels of the head. Elmer and Alyce Green, two innovators in the field of biofeedback training, taught sufferers of migraines to raise the temperature of their hands, which dilated hand blood vessels and diminished the dilation of the vessels of the head.

The Current Status of Biofeedback

The use of biofeedback training has gained increased acceptance by the medical profession. It currently plays an important role in behavioral medicine. For the past ten years the American Medical Assocation has offered biofeedback workshops at annual meetings. A growing area of interest to many people, it is a technique that has demonstrated success but that has many unanswered questions requiring further research.

How to Find a Biofeedback Practitioner

As mentioned earlier, biofeedback is not a treatment but a process of learning. Thus, its professional use is based on knowledge of social and biological factors combined with teaching skill. No specific licensing procedures exist for the certification of biofeedback practitioners. It is used by doctors, social workers, dentists, psychologists, physical therapists, occupational therapists, as well as a variety of other health care practitioners. As Elmer Green states, "biofeedback is not a miracle cure, it is a tool for all professions."

CHIROPRACTIC

Physical changes that accompany the aging process often plague older people with vague "aches and pains," and the quality of our lives can be deeply affected by this chronic discomfort. If a person's family health care practitioner cannot relieve pain, the sufferer often and understandably seeks other nontraditional sources of relief—often from a chiropractor.

Chiropractic intervention claims to treat and manage headaches, chronic pain, rheumatoid and osteoarthritis, allergies, nervous tension, migraine headaches, lower back problems, disc syndromes, strains and sprains, fatigue, postural defects, functional disorders of internal organs, hypertension, as well as symptoms related to menopause.

What Is Chiropractic?

Chiropractic has been defined as: "a system of manipulative treatment which teaches that all diseases are caused by impingement on spinal nerves and can be corrected by spinal adjustments."

Chiropractic healing is geared toward the maintenance of the integrity of the nervous system, because it maintains that the nervous system controls the function of all organs, muscles, and tissues of the body.

The spinal cord, which is housed within the spine, is considered to be the "switchboard" of the nervous system. Nerve pathways pass from the brain through the spinal cord, to deliver impulses or messages to all the organs of the body. These impulses leave the spinal cord through the spinal vertebrae (the bones of the spine). If the spinal column is misaligned, it can interfere with this normal communication network, resulting in an imbalance in the body's normal functioning. Thus, the primary therapeutic tool of chiropractors is manipulation of the spine to correct misalignment.

According to Daniel David Palmer, the man most often credited with the discovery of chiropractic in the late nineteenth century: "Illness is essentially functional and becomes organic only as an end process."

Today, most chiropractors engender a wholistic approach to healing which relies on neither drugs nor surgery. They also recognize the effect that external factors can have on the body's state of balance. For instance, some chiropractors also work with their patients' nutrition, stress reduction, and other aspects of illness prevention and health maintenance.

A visit to a chiropractor (who *must* be licensed) should entail an initial health assessment to inform the practitioner as to whether the patient could benefit from chiropractic intervention. If a serious problem (e.g., certain cardiovascular conditions or malignancies) are suspected, a referral to a medical doctor must be made.

Older people, who must be confronted with a variety of conditions that effect the musculoskeletal system, can benefit from chiropractic treatment providing they have no serious health problems that require traditional medical supervision.

If you do decide to see a chiropractor, it is important that you inform your health care practitioner of the treatment you are receiving. In many instances, chiropractic should be used only in conjunction with more traditional treatments offered by health care practitioners. Unfortunately, most chiropractors function autonomously and are thus divorced from the traditional medical system.

Since the inception of chiropractic almost one hundred years ago, organized medicine has been lobbying against the profession. However, within the past ten years there has been increased public acceptance as well as legal recognition and licensing of chiropractors.

Insurance policies regarding reimbursement for chiropractic services vary from state to state, although most policies do provide coverage. In addition, Medicare payments for chiropractic services were made to persons over 65 in 1974.

How to Choose a Chiropractor

Find a *licensed* chiropractor that you trust so that you can easily ask questions about the treatments you receive.

Professional chiropractors are listed in the Yellow Pages of the telephone directory, and every state has a local chapter of the American Chiropractic Association from which you can get referrals.

MASSAGE

Massage, a form of "therapeutic touch" or reaching out to another person through touch, can soothe the mind and body, relieve stress and tension, and stimulate health.

Although massage as a form of healing and prevention has been growing in popularity in the 1980s, it is one of the oldest forms of healing, having been practiced for thousands of years. Hippocrates, a Greek physician living in the fourth century B.C., who is referred to as the "Father of Medicine," believed that all physicians should be experienced in "friction."

Massage has been used for the following purposes:

a) to alleviate stress and tension
b) to provide a drugless sedative effect

c) for treatment of headaches, arthritis, circulatory problems, and constipation
d) for strengthening of weak muscles
e) to help someone simply to feel good

Many different types of massage are practiced in the United States today, but common to all is the application of hands to manipulate parts of the body by pressure, kneading movements, friction, vibration, and percussion. Massage increases the circulation of blood, oxygen supply, and important nutrients in the massaged area.

These are some of the more popular forms of massage practiced today:

1. *Swedish massage*—a practice developed by Per Henrik Ling in the early nineteenth century stimulates the skin, the nervous system, and the muscles, and helps to alleviate pains and tension. As practiced today, Swedish massage is used both in medical as well as in nonmedical settings.

Techniques used for Swedish massage involve:

a) *effleurage*—a stroking movement
b) *petrissage*—manipulation of the muscle tissues
c) *percussion*—beating and pounding
d) *running vibration*—the fingertips following the course of the nerves

e) *friction*—to help restore mobility to joint surfaces

2. *Shiatsu*—a Japanese system of massage based on ancient Chinese teachings which applies finger pressure to points on the body known as *tsubos*. These points correspond to the meridians of the body. This pressure stimulates the flow of *ki*, or body energy. It is interesting to note that the actual points on the body where pressure is applied are not always the points where the person is experiencing the pain.

3. *Reflexology*—also based on techniques of ancient Chinese origin which maintain that the feet are important to the health of the rest of the body, and that each organ of the body corresponds to a specific point on each foot. When pressure is applied to these points, areas of blocked energy flow caused by the accumulation of various acids, waste products, and utilized calcium, are released.

When Massage Should Not Be Used

As with all alternatives to traditional care, massage should never replace the services of a health care practitioner. Such conditions as high fever, pain associated with an infection, hemorrhage, thrombosis, phlebitis, varicose veins, fractures, diarrhea, jaundice, or abdominal masses can be complicated by massage, and require medical treatment.

How to Find a Massage Therapist

Some massage therapists practice in Y's, health spas, and saunas. If you live in an area where there is a massage institute, it may be able to provide referrals for local practitioners. Some massage therapists are licensed by the AMTA (American Massage Therapy Association).

OSTEOPATHY

The basic underlying principles of osteopathy are based on the mobilization of the body's own forces to stimulate healing and to preserve health. Osteopaths diagnose and treat numerous health problems through *palpation* (examination by application of the hands or fingers to the external surface of the body) and *spinal manipulation*. However, osteopaths have integrated many of the more traditional approaches to medicine into their practices. For instance, D.O.'s (Doctors of Osteopathy) also utilize drugs and surgical procedures as part of their practice.

Looking for an answer to the question, What is an osteopathic physician? we find no simple reply. Even within the field of osteopathic medicine, there is little agreement as to the exact definition of osteopathy.

A 1981 survey of practicing D.O.'s geared toward understanding the characteristics of osteopathy stated that practitioners felt that their profession was a discipline related to "body unity, the capacity for self-regulation and the interdependence of structure and function."

The American Osteopathic Association states that: "osteopathic medicine focuses special attention on the biological mechanisms by which the musculoskeletal system, through the nervous and circulatory systems, interacts with all the body organs and systems in both health and disease."

Osteopathic medicine is not necessarily considered an alternative to, but rather as a complement to, medical care as it exists today. It considers itself "something more—not something else."

HISTORY AND PHILOSOPHY:

The principles of osteopathic medicine are derived from Dr. Andrew Taylor Still, who practiced medicine in the 1800s. Dr. Still, an early supporter of women's and civil rights, was not satisfied with the quality, theory, and practice of the medicine of his time. He believed that the medical profession focused too heavily on the treatment of disease rather than viewing the body as a functional unit. Dr. Still's dissatisfaction with traditional medical treatment led to his contribution to the development of osteopathy.

Dr. Still believed that the human body functions properly when it is mechanically sound and that the body has the ability to cure itself. An understanding of the relationship between treatment of illness and spinal manipulation is paramount to the osteopathic discipline.

Originally, the practice of osteopathy was not

readily accepted by more traditional medical practitioners. In the late nineteenth century, it was considered by many to be a form of medical quackery. The situation today has changed quite dramatically, as the American Medical Association has publicly accepted the practice of osteopathy.

Present-day Osteopathy

Today almost 90 percent of osteopathic physicians are currently in general family practice. D.O.'s are participants in the Medicare and Medicaid programs, as well as in private health insurance programs. This has eased some of the burden created by the growing specialization of health care which has created a severe shortage of primary health care practitioners, especially in rural areas.

Osteopaths are licensed in all fifty states and serve as principal health care practitioners in some parts of the country, particularly in rural areas and small cities.

Licensing laws for osteopathic physicians are the responsibility of state licensing boards. Thus, standards and requirements vary from state to state. However, requirements in all states are quite similar, and these basically state that osteopaths can provide the same services as those provided by M.D.'s.

D.O.'s receive intensive training in anatomy, physiology, chemistry, pathology, microbiology, immunology, and pharmacology.

It is very important to find a practitioner with whom you feel a sense of warmth and trust, regardless of whether he or she is an M.D., a D.O., or any other type of health care practitioner. For further information on osteopathic medicine, you can contact the divisional Osteopathic Society in your state. Every state, with the exception of Alaska and Mississippi, has such a society.

THERAPEUTIC TOUCH

Most of us have experienced the calming effect that touching or being touched by another person can have. "Therapeutic touch" is a healing technique utilized by some nurses as well as other health care practitioners and spiritual healers involving the supposed transfer of energy from one individual to another.

Therapeutic touch was introduced into modern-day health care, specifically to the nursing profession, by Dolores Krieger, who is herself a nurse. Krieger studied the ancient practice of "the laying on of hands," a technique used for healing in many ancient cultures, including early Indian, Tibetan, Egyptian, and Roman and other European civilizations. Krieger's studies of the spiritual as well as scientific frameworks of the discipline attempted to understand the relationship between a healer and an ill subject.

Central to an understanding of "the laying on of hands," and thus to the practice of therapeutic touch, is the Eastern concept of *prana*, which is not easily defined or understood through traditional

Western thinking and assumptions about the world. *Prana* is the flow of "life energy," in essence the "life breath." Krieger believes that *prana* is closely related to, and can be compared with, the Western concept of the oxygen molecule. Health is considered to be a state of being which is marked by an overabundance of *prana*, whereas illness usually represents a deficit or an expression of an imbalance in the flow of energy through one's body.

The Process

Therapeutic touch relies on neither drugs nor machines but is a meditative communication between two people for the purpose of repatterning energies that might have caused tension, pain, and disease.

An initial assessment of the areas of imbalance throughout a person's body is followed by treatment which helps to redirect energy, or *prana*. The healer will first assess her subject by "listening" with her hands. She will use her hands to scan the subject's body for areas of tension and/or heat. After this "listening" phase, the healer will continue to use her hands to redirect the subject's energies to alleviate these tensions and to restore balance. The healer first "centers" herself so as to focus on the subject's energy flow, without any distraction.

Contemporary scientific studies have indicated the effective uses of therapeutic touch in some healing practices.

Practitioners

Therapeutic touch is used by some nurses as well as other health care practitioners and spiritual healers and is taught in some nursing programs in the United States.

It is important that you ask a nurse or other health care practitioner to explain the method to you in language that you can understand.

APPENDICES

APPENDIX ONE
Advocacy—Agencies and Programs

1. Specifically concerned with older women:
   A. The Older Women's League (OWL)
      3800 Harrison St.
      Oakland, CA 94611 (Check your telephone
      directory for local chapters.)

      Organized in 1981 as an outgrowth of the
      National Organization of Women (NOW)
      Mini Conference on Older Women, prior to
      the 1981 White House Conference on Ag-
      ing.

   B. Displaced Homemakers Center, Inc.
      5000 MacArthur Boulevard
      Oakland, CA 94619

      For further information see Appendix 7 on
      money management.

2. General:
   A. American Association of Retired Persons
      1909 K St. N.W.
      Washington, DC 20049

B. National Association of Retired Federal Employees
1533 New Hampshire Circle, N.W.
Washington, DC 20036

C. The Gray Panthers
3635 Chestnut St.
Philadelphia, PA 19164

D. National Caucus and Center on Black Aged
1424 K St. N.W.
Washington, DC 20005

E. National Council on the Aging, Inc.
600 Maryland Ave. S.W.
Washington, DC 20002 (Public Policy Center)

F. National Council of Senior Citizens
925 Fifteenth St. N.W.
Washington, DC 20005 (Lobbying organization)

G. National Interfaith Coalition on Aging
289 South Hall St.
Athens, GA. 30601

H. Senior Political Action Committee (PAC)
1900 M St. N.W.
Washington, DC 20036

I. Urban Elderly Coalition
600 Maryland Ave.
Washington, DC 20036

APPENDIX TWO
Education—Agencies and Programs

A. The Adult Education Association of the
   U.S.A.
   1201 Sixteenth St. N.W., Suite 230
   Washington, D.C. 20036

B. Elder Hostel
   100 Boylston St.
   Boston, MA 02116

   Network of colleges and universities offering low-cost residential programs during the
   summer for persons 60 and over, featuring
   noncredit courses, largely in the liberal arts.

C. Institute of Lifetime Learning
   American Association of Retired Persons
      (AARP)
   1909 K St. N.W.
   Washington, DC 20049

   Extension courses cosponsored by local
   educational institutions, free or reduced tu-

ition for older people. Local chapters nationwide.

D. Institute for Retired Professionals
New School for Social Research
66 W. 12th St.
New York, NY 10011

For retired professionals and executives. Offers flexible curriculum.

E. National Council on the Aging, Inc.
600 Maryland Ave. S.W.
Washington, DC 20002

   1) Senior Center Humanities Program
Learning units available for senior center programs.
   2) The Center on Arts and the Aging

F. National Home Study Council
1601 17th St. N.W.
Washington, DC 20009

Directory of accredited schools offering home study courses.

G. National University Continuing Education Association
One DuPont Circle N.W.
Suite 360
Washington, DC 20036

List of universities offering independent study programs.

In addition to colleges, universities, and senior centers, many public school systems offer programs and courses for retired persons. Call your local school's Office of Adult and Continuing Education for information.

APPENDIX THREE
Employment—Agencies and Programs

A. American Association of Retired Persons (AARP)
   1909 K St. N.W.
   Washington, DC 20049

B. Mature Temps, Inc.
   1114 Avenue of the Americas
   New York, NY 10036 (Local offices)

   Senior community service employment program

C. National Caucus and Center on Black Aged
   1424 K St. N.W.
   Washington, DC 20005 (Job bank center)

D. National Council on the Aging, Inc.
   600 Maryland Ave, S.W.
   Washington, DC 20002

E. National Council of Senior Citizens
925 15th St. N.W.
Washington, DC 20005 (Senior aides program)

F. Title V—Older Americans Act
For information, contact local Office for the Aging.

See also Appendix 15, "Volunteer Opportunities," under ACTION for low-paying, part-time government employment. Local communities also have employment opportunities. Check with your nearest Office for the Aging.

APPENDIX FOUR
Health Care

1. General
   A. National Association for Human Development
   1620 I St. N.W.
   Washington, DC 20006

   Health and social services for persons over 65. Offers self-help workshops on retirement, physical fitness, preventive health care, nutrition, and vocational training.

B. National Women's Health Network
224 7th St. S.W.
Washington, DC 20024

Concerned with women's health *vis-à-vis* the health care system.

2. Government Food Programs
   A. Food Stamp Program
   Food coupons which can be used in retail food stores participating in the Food Stamp Program are distributed directly to eligible households. Administered by the State Department of Social Services in most states, the program is designed to improve the diet of members of low-income households by supplementing food-purchasing ability. Most grocery stores are authorized to accept food stamps.

   Eligibility for food stamps is determined on the basis of financial need, assessed by considering the number of persons living in a household, the income of the household, and the resources and assets available to members of the household.

   For older disabled people who are unable to buy and prepare their own food, food stamps can be used to pay for delivery of food by authorized meal delivery programs. In addition, older people are entitled to use food stamps to purchase meals in settings providing communal dining for the elderly.

Through the Food Stamp Program, individuals can also receive free pamphlets pertaining to food stamps, and to nutrition in general, such as:

1) *Characteristics of Food Stamps Households*
2) *How to Apply For and Use Food Stamps*
3) *Building a Better Diet*
4) *Tips for Non-Profit Communal Dining Facilities*

The above pamphlets can be obtained by writing to your regional Food Stamp office. For information on where your regional Food Stamp office is, you can write to:

Food and Nutrition Service
US Department of Agriculture
Alexandria, VA 22302

If you are interested in applying for food stamps, contact your local Department of Social Services to make an appointment. The telephone directory listing is usually found under "State Government Offices."

When you call for an appointment, be sure to ask what types of documentation you need to take with you for your first interview.

If you are interested in more information on food stamps, write to:

Food Stamp Research Action Center (FRAC)
2011 I St. N.W.
Washington, DC 20006

B. Nutrition Services Programs

A variety of nutrition programs exist in local communities which provide older people with low-cost nutritious meals and with education relating to maintaining a healthful diet. Such programs are authorized under the Older Americans Act of 1965, Title III, Part C, through the U.S. Office of Human Development Services, Department of Health and Human Services, 200 Independence Ave. S.W., Washington, DC 20201.

People age 60 and over are eligible for nutrition programs. Meals are generally served in a congregate setting or delivered to homes or apartments (a service sometimes referred to as "Meals on Wheels").

Nutrition programs are usually offered through churches, synagogues, senior centers, schools, or other community agencies.

If you are interested in learning where in your area you can become involved in a nutrition program, or how you can go about receiving a home-delivered meal, contact your local Department for the Aging, political representative, or social service agency.

3. Nutrition Charts

RECOMMENDED DIETARY ALLOWANCES Differences Between Younger and Older Age Groups[1]			
FEMALES 55 kg.–120 lbs. 163 cm.–64 in. Age Group in Years			
Substance	23–50	51+	76+
Energy (kcal)	2000	1800	1600
Energy range	1600–2400	1400–2200	1200–2000
Protein (gm)	44	44	
Vitamin A (mcg RE)[2]	800	800	
Vitamin D (mcg)[3]	5	5	
Vitamin E (mαTE)[4]	8	8	
Ascorbic Acid (mg)	60	60	
Thiamine (mg)	1.0	1.0	
Riboflavin (mg)	1.2	1.2	
Niacin (mg NE)[5]	13	13	
Vitamin B-6 (mg)	2.0	2.0	
Folacin (mcg)	400	400	
Vitamin B-12 (mcg)	3	3	
Calcium (mg)	800	800	
Phosphorus (mg)	800	800	
Magnesium (mg)	300	300	
Iron (mg)	18	10	
Zinc (mg)	15	15	
Iodine (mcg)	150	150	

1. Source: Recommended Dietary Allowances, 9th Revised Edition, National Academy of Sciences, Washington, DC, 1980. Full text is available from: Office of Publications
    National Academy of Sciences
    2101 Constitution Avenue N.W.
    Washington, DC 20418
2. Retinol equivalents. 1 RE = 1 mcg retinol or 6 mcg beta-carotene.
3. A cholecalciferol. 10 mcg cholecalciferol = 400 I.U. vitamin D.
4. αTocopherol equivalents. 1 mgα-αtocopherol = 1 TE.
5. Niacin equivalents. 1 NE = 1 mg niacin or 60 mg dietary tryptophan.

3. Nutrition Charts (continued)

APPROXIMATE ENERGY EXPENDITURE BY A 150-POUND PERSON IN VARIOUS ACTIVITIES[1]	
Activity	**Calories per hour**
Lying down or sleeping	80
Sitting	100
Driving an automobile	120
Standing	140
Domestic work	180
Walking, 2½ mph	210
Bicycling, 5½ mph	210
Gardening	220
Golf; lawn mowing (power mower)	250
Bowling	270
Walking, 3¾ mph	300
Swimming, ¼ mph	300
Square dancing, volleyball, roller skating	350
Wood chopping or sawing	400
Tennis	420
Skiing, 10 mph	600
Squash and handball	600
Bicycling, 13 mph	660
Running, 10 mph	900

1. Source: Based on material prepared by Robert E. Johnson, M.D., Ph.D., and colleagues, Univ. of Illinois.

Height (with 2-in. heel shoes)	Weight in Pounds According to Frame (in Indoor Clothing)		
DESIRABLE WEIGHTS—AGES 25 AND OVER[1] **WOMEN**			
Feet, Inches	**Small Frame**	**Medium Frame**	**Large Frame**
4' 10"	92–98	96–107	104–119
4' 11"	94–101	98–110	106–122
5' 0"	96–104	101–113	109–125
5' 1"	99–107	104–116	112–128
5' 2"	102–110	107–119	115–131
5' 3"	105–113	110–122	118–134
5' 4"	108–116	113–126	121–138
5' 5"	111–119	116–130	125–142
5' 6"	114–123	120–135	129–146
5' 7"	118–127	124–139	133–150
5' 8"	122–131	128–143	137–154
5' 9"	126–135	132–147	141–158
5' 10"	130–140	136–151	145–163
5' 11"	134–144	140–155	149–168
6' 0"	138–148	144–159	153–173

1. Source: Based on material by Metropolitan Life.

APPENDIX FIVE
Housing—Agencies and Programs

A. Cooperative League of the USA
   1828 L St. N.W.
   Washington, DC 20036

A national confederation of cooperatives which provides its members with educational materials, newsletters, and information exchange relating to the development of cooperatives. The league promotes self-help to older people and in particular provides information and technical assistance on cooperatives and how to use them in areas such as housing, health, consumer goods, recreation, nutrition, etc.

B. International Center for Social Gerontology
   600 Maryland Ave. S.W.
   Washington, DC 20002

   Promotes activities for older people geared toward generating more and higher-quality housing and related services. The center makes available an extensive collection of material and information, particularly in the area of housing.

C. National Council on the Aging, Inc.
   Housing Corporation
   600 Maryland Ave. S.W.
   Washington, DC 20002

D. US Office of Housing and Urban Development (HUD)
   451 Seventh St. S.W.
   Washington, DC 20410

1) The Program Information Center
   A federal agency which provides information and referral to individuals and groups on issues related to housing. The center assists older people in areas such as housing availability and subsidies and provides information to groups interested in developing housing programs in their local communities.

2) Congregate Housing Services Program Office of Multi-Family Development Housing
   Provides grants to organizations initiating projects designed to provide housing to elderly populations. Specifically, projects must meet the following objectives:

   a) to prevent premature or unnecessary institutionalization of the elderly;
   b) to provide a variety of innovative approaches for the delivery of meals and nonmedical supportive services;
   c) to fill gaps in existing service systems to ensure the availability of funding for meals and appropriate services.

To receive a grant application, or further information, write to the Congregate Housing Program.

3) Housing Assistance Program (Section 8)

Provides aid to low-income families in obtaining decent, safe, and sanitary housing. The program provides housing assistance to participating private owners and Public Housing agencies on behalf of eligible tenants. Assisted families are expected to contribute at least 30% of their adjusted family income toward rent.

Individuals eligible for this program include families whose income does not exceed 50% of the average income for a particular geographic area as determined by HUD.

For further information, contact HUD, listed under "United States Government" in your telephone directory.

4) Housing Loan Program (Section 202)

A loan program designed to provide rental or cooperative housing for the aged and/or disabled through non-profit organizations providing a capital investment of one-half to one percent of the mortgage amount of a proposed housing facility with a maximum of up to $10,000.

APPENDIX SIX
Legal Resources—Agencies and Programs

A. Administration on Aging
   US Department of Health and Human Services
   200 Independence Ave. S.W.
   Washington, DC 20201

B. National Lawyers Guild
   853 Broadway
   New York, NY 10003

C. National Legal Aid and Defender Association
   1625 K St. N.W.
   Washington, DC 20006

D. National Senior Citizens Law Center
   1424 16th St. N.W.
   Washington, DC 20036

Some private law firms specialize in counseling older people. For information, consult your local bar association.

APPENDIX SEVEN
Money Management—Agencies and Programs

A. American Association of Retired Persons (AARP)
   Tax Aide Program
   1909 K St. N.W.
   Washington, DC 20049

   Provides assistance to older people in filing federal tax returns, information on particular tax credits specifically designed for older people, and information on tax breaks for low-income people over age 65 who are selling their homes. In addition, this organization also recruits older people as volunteers to provide tax-aid services to others.

B. Displaced Homemakers
   5000 MacArthur Blvd.
   Oakland, CA 94619

   A national organization which advocates for displaced homemakers throughout the country; serves as a clearinghouse for information pertaining to displaced homemakers; has regional and statewide chapters. Newsletter is available for a $3.00 fee by writing to the organization at the above address.

APPENDIX EIGHT
Nursing Homes—Agencies and Programs

1. Organizations
   A. Administration on Aging
      US Department of Health and Human Services
      Nursing Home Ombudsman Program
      200 Independence Ave. S.W.
      Washington, DC 20201

      Organizes statewide advocacy units to investigate complaints about nursing home care; and then works to resolve problems on behalf of nursing home residents. For information, call State Office for the Aging.

   B. American Association of Homes for the Aging
      1050 17th St. N.W.
      Suite 770
      Washington, DC 20036

      Provides information to the general public on how to choose a nursing home.

   C. American College of Nursing Home Administrators
      4650 East-West Highway
      Bethesda, MD 20014

      A professional association whose members

are concerned with education and research related to nursing home care.

D. American Health Care Association
   1200 15th St. N.W.
   Washington, DC 20005

A federation of 47 state long-term care associations representing providers (owners and administrators) of nursing homes. The federation is also involved with monitoring pending legislative issues affecting older people, as well as providing a variety of written material to consumers of nursing home care.

Write to the American Health Care Association for copies of their pamphlets. Two pamphlets that might be of particular interest are:

1) *Thinking About a Nursing Home*
2) *Welcome to Our Nursing Home*

E. Friends and Relatives of the Institutionalized Aged (FRIA)
   440 E. 26th St.
   New York, NY 10010

A New York-based membership organization designed to advocate for the needs of residents of long-term care facilities. A booklet on nursing home advocacy, including information on how to choose a nursing home, can be obtained by writing to FRIA. Ask for *A Consumer's Guide to Nursing Home Care in New York.*

F. US Department of Health and Human Services

Has the responsibility to monitor and evaluate nursing homes according to standards set by State and Federal Nursing Home Codes. Complaints about nursing homes can be reported to the Department, which has the responsibility to respond to such complaints through the State Health Department.

Inspection reports of all nursing homes, available at Departments of Health nationwide, are public information. Consumers of nursing home care, whether they be friends, relatives, or concerned citizens, are encouraged to review these inspection reports.

The Department also sends copies of inspection reports to individual nursing home facilities. Administrators are expected to allow consumers to review these reports upon request.

For information on how to review inspection reports for nursing homes in your area, call the State Department of Health and Human Services, listed under "State Government" in your telephone directory.

2. How to Choose a Nursing Home

When considering a nursing home placement for yourself or a friend or relative, it is important to "shop around" for the facility best suited for the particular individual. Assessment of the appropriate place depends on the needs of the person who will be living there.

Some important things to look for, think about, and question are listed here:

1) Are there handrails on the walls?
2) Are there ramps for wheelchairs so that handicapped people can go outside?
3) Is the home in a convenient location for friends and relatives to visit?
4) Do you detect an odor of urine when you enter the facility, or in the area where residents live?
5) Do you observe the staff interacting with the residents?
6) Are there smoke detectors on the ceilings?
7) Are residents involved in activities, or are the activity rooms empty?
8) Do the rooms appear to be clean?
9) Is there a Patient Bill of Rights hanging on the wall in the front lobby?
10) Does the kitchen appear to be clean?
11) Is the menu posted outside the dining room?

It is important to note that the outside appearance of a nursing home does not always indicate the quality of care received inside. Based on the above key points, combined with your own sense of judgment, try to select a nursing home that you feel comfortable with.

APPENDIX NINE
Organizations—Aging and General

1. Government Agencies and Committees
   A. Administration on Aging
      US Department of Health and Human Services
      200 Independence Ave. S.W.
      Washington, DC 20201

   B. National Association of State Units on Aging
      600 Maryland Ave. S.W.
      Washington, DC 20024

   C. National Institute on Aging
      National Institutes of Health
      US Department of Health and Human Services
      9000 Rockville Pike
      Bethesda, MD 20014 (Research on Aging)

   D. Select Committee on Aging
      US House of Representatives
      Washington, DC 20515

E. Social Security Administration
   (see local offices under "US Government" in
      your telephone directory)

F. Special Committee on Aging
   US Senate
   Washington, DC 20510

G. Veterans Administration
   (See local offices under "US Government"
      in your telephone directory)

2. State Agencies on Aging

Alabama
Commission on Aging
State Capitol
Montgomery, AL
   36130

Alaska
Division of Adult and
   Aging Services
Pouch H-OIC
Juneau, AK 99811

Arizona
Aging and Adult
   Administration
1400 West Washing-
   ton St.
P.O. Box 6123
Phoenix, AZ 85005

Arkansas
Office on Aging and
   Adult Services
Dept. of Social and
   Rehabilitation
   Services
Donaghey Bldg.,
   Room I031S
Little Rock, AR
   77201

California
Department of Aging
918 J St.
Sacramento, CA 95814

Colorado
Division of Services
   for the Aging

Department of Social
Services, Room 503
1575 Sherman St.
Denver, CO 80220

Connecticut
Department on Aging
80 Washington St.,
Room 312
Hartford, CT 06115

Delaware
Division of Aging
Dept. of Health and
Social Services
1901 North DuPont
Highway
Newcastle, DE 19720

District of Columbia
Office on Aging
Office of the Mayor
1424 K St. N.W.
Washington, DC
20005

Florida
Program Office of Ag-
ing and Adult
Services
Dept. of Health and
Rehabilitation
Services
1323 Winewood Blvd.
Tallahassee, FL 32301

Georgia
Department of Aging
Section
Department of Hu-
man Resources
618 Ponce de Leon
Ave. N.E.
Atlanta, GA 30308

Hawaii
Executive Office on
Aging
Office of the Governor
State of Hawaii
1149 Bethel St., Room
307
Honolulu, HI 96813

Idaho
Idaho Office on Aging
State House
Boise, ID 83720

Illinois
Department on Aging
421 East Capital
Avenue
Springfield, IL 62706

Indiana
Commission on the
Aging and Aged
215 North Senate Ave.
Indianapolis, IN
46202

Iowa
Commission on Aging
415 W. 10th St.
Jewett Bldg.
Des Moines, IA 50319

Kansas
Department on Aging
610 W. 10th St.
Topeka, KS 66612

Kentucky
Division for Aging
  Services
Department of Hu-
  man Services
DHR Bldg., 6th Floor
275 E. Main St.
Frankfort, KY 40601

Louisiana
Office of Elderly
  Affairs
P.O. Box 44282
Capital Station
Baton Rouge, LA
  70804

Maine
Bureau of Maine's El-
  derly Community
  Services Unit
Department of Hu-
  man Services
State House

Augusta, ME 04333

Maryland
Office on Aging
State Office Bldg.
301 W. Preston St.
Baltimore, MD 21201

Massachusetts
Department of Elder
  Affairs
88 Chauncy St., 5th
  Floor
Boston, MA 02111

Michigan
Offices of Services to
  the Aging
300 E. Michigan Ave.
P.O. Box 30026
Lansing, MI 48909

Minnesota
Minnesota Board on
  Aging
Metro Square Bldg.,
  Room 204
7th and Robert Streets
St. Paul, MN 55101

Mississippi
Mississippi Council on
  Aging
Executive Bldg., Suite
  301

802 N. State St.
Jackson, MS 39201

Missouri
Division on Aging
Dept. of Social
 Services
Broadway State
P.O. Box 570
Jefferson City, MO
 65101

Montana
Community Services
 Division
P.O. Box 4210
Helena, MT 59601

Nebraska
Commission on Aging
P.O. Box 95044
301 Centennial Mall
 South
Lincoln, NE 68509

Nevada
Division of Aging
Dept. of Human
 Resources
505 E. King St.
Kinkead Bldg., Room
 101
Carson City, NV
 88710

New Hampshire
Council on Aging
14 Depot St.
Concord, NH 03301

New Jersey
Division on Aging
Dept. of Community
 Affairs
P.O. Box 2768
363 W. State St.
Trenton, NJ 08625

New Mexico
State Agency on
 Aging
440 St. Michael's Dr.
Chamisa Hills Bldg.
Santa Fe, NM 87503

New York
Office for the Aging
New York State Exec-
 utive Dept.
Empire State Plaza
Agency Bldg. #2
Albany, NY 12223

North Carolina
North Carolina De-
 partment of Human
 Resources
Division on Aging
708 Hillsborough St.
Raleigh, NC 27608

North Dakota
Aging Services
Social Services Board
   of North Dakota
State Capitol Building
Bismarck, ND 58505

Ohio
Commission on Aging
50 W. Broad St., 9th
   Floor
Columbus, OH 43215

Oklahoma
Special Unit on Aging
Dept. of Human
   Services
P.O. Box 25352
Oklahoma City, OK
   73125

Oregon
Office of Elderly
   Affairs
Human Resources
   Department
772 Commercial St.
   S.E.
Salem, OR 97310

Pennsylvania
Department of Aging
Room 404
Finance Bldg.
Harrisburg, PA 17120

Rhode Island
Department of Elderly
   Affairs
79 Washington St.
Providence, RI 02903

South Carolina
Commission on Aging
915 Main St.
Columbia, SC 29201

South Dakota
Office on Aging
South Dakota Dept.
   of Social Services
State Office Bldg.
Illinois St.
Pierre, SD 57501

Tennessee
Commission on Aging
703 Tennessee Bldg.
535 Church St.
Nashville, TN 37219

Texas
Governor's Committee
   on Aging
210 Martin Springs
   Rd., 5th Floor
P.O. Box 12786, Capi-
   tal Station
Austin, TX 78704

Utah
Division on Aging
Dept. of Social
  Services
150 West North Tem-
  ple St.
Box 2500
Salt Lake City, UT
  84102

Vermont
Office on Aging
Agency on Human
  Services
State Office Bldg.
Montpelier, VT 05602

Virginia
Office on Aging
830 E. Main St., Suite
  950
Richmond, VA 23219

Washington
Bureau of Aging and
  Adult Services
Dept. of Social and
  Health Services OB-
  43G
Olympia, WA 98504

West Virginia
Commission on Aging
State Capitol
Charleston, WV 25305

Wisconsin
Bureau on Aging
One W. Wilson St.,
  Room 685
Madison, WI 53702

Wyoming
Commission on Aging
720 W. 18th St.
Cheyenne, WY 82002

*US Unincorporated
Territories*
American Samoa
Territorial Aging
  Program
Office of the Governor
Pago Pago, AS 96799

Guam
Office of Aging
Social Services Dept.
  of Public Health
Government of Guam
P.O. Box 2618
Agana, GU 96910

Puerto Rico
Gericulture
  Commission
Department of Social
  Services
P.O. Box 11368
Santurce, PR 00908

Trust Territory of the
Pacific Islands
Office of Elderly
  Programs
Government of TTPI
Civic Center, Susupe
Saipan, Northern
  Mariana Island
  96950

Virgin Islands
Commission on Aging
P.O. Box 539
Charlotte Amalie
St. Thomas, VI 00801

3. Nonprofit Agencies on Aging
   A. American Association of Retired Persons
      (AARP)
      1909 K St. N.W.
      Washington, DC 20049 (Local chapters)

      Age Discrimination Project
      Anti-Crime Guide
      Institute of Lifetime Learning
      Mature Temps
      Senior Community Service Employment
        Program
      Tax Aide Program
      Widowed Persons Service

   B. The Gray Panthers
      3635 Chestnut St.
      Philadelphia, PA 19104 (Local chapters)

   C. International Senior Citizens Association,
      Inc.
      11753 Wilshire Blvd.
      Los Angeles, CA 90025

D. National Association for Human Development
1620 I St. N.W.
Washington, DC 20006

E. National Association of Retired Federal Employees
1533 New Hampshire Ave. N.W.
Washington, DC 20036

F. National Council on the Aging, Inc.
600 Maryland Ave. S.W.
Washington, DC 20002

National Medical Resource Center on Aging
National Institute of Senior Citizens
Senior Center Humanities Program
National Institute of Work and Retirement
   Pre-retirement Planning Project
NCOA Housing Corp.
National Voluntary Organization for Independent Living for the Aging
Public Policy Center
Center on Arts and the Aging
Intergenerational Services Program
List of NCOA Publications

G. National Caucus and Center on Black Aged
1424 K St. N.W.
Washington, DC 20005 (Job bank center)

H. National Council of Senior Citizens
   925 15th St. N.W.
   Washington, DC 20005

I. National Interfaith Coalition on Aging
   289 South Hull St.
   Athens, GA 30601

J. Older Women's League (OWL)
   3800 Harrison St.
   Oakland, CA 94611

K. Urban Elderly Coalition
   600 Maryland Ave.
   Washington, DC 20036

4. Agencies on Sexuality

   A. Educational Foundation for Human Sexuality
      Montclair State College
      Upper Montclair, NJ 07043

   B. National Institute of Mental Health
      5600 Fishers Lane
      Bethesda, MD 20857

   C. Sex Information Education Council of the US (SIECUS)
      80 Fifth Ave.
      New York, NY 10011

APPENDIX TEN
Organizations—Disease-Related

1. Alcoholism
   A. Alcohol and Drug Problems Association of North America
      1101 15th St. N.W., Suite 204
      Washington, DC 20005

      Disseminates information on addiction, encourages legislation designed to control alcohol and drug abuse, and sponsors drug and alcohol treatment and referral centers.

   B. Alcoholics Anonymous
      General Services Office
      468 Park Ave. South
      New York, NY 10016

      AA self-help groups are located throughout the world. For more information, request the brochure entitled *This is AA* from the above address.

   C. National Council on Alcoholism, Inc.
      733 Third Ave.
      New York, NY 10017

      A volunteer-supported organization, working for the prevention and control of alcoholism through programs of public and professional education, the NCA publishes literature on alcoholism and its treatment; sponsors community alcohol rehabilitation programs; and supports research on the causes, prevention, and treatment of alcoholism.

D. National Institute on Alcohol Abuse and Alcoholism
US Department of Health and Human Services
Public Health Service
Alcohol, Drug Abuse, and Mental Health Administration
5600 Fishers Lane
Rockville, MD 20857 (National clearinghouse for alcohol information)

E. Women for Sobriety, Inc.
Box 618
Quakertown, PA 18951

An international organization helping women with drinking problems to achieve sobriety and a fulfilling way of life.

2. Alzheimer's Disease
A. Alzheimer's Disease and Related Disorders Association (ADRDA)
360 N. Michigan Ave.
Chicago, IL 60601

B. National Institute of Neurological and Com-

municative Disorders and Stroke
Office of Scientific and Health Reports
Bldg. 31, Room 8A08
National Institutes of Health
9000 Rockville Pike
Bethesda, MD 20014

3. Arthritis
   A. Arthritis Foundation
      3400 Peachtree Rd. N.E.
      Atlanta, GA 30326 (Local chapters)

      A voluntary health association dedicated to finding the cause of arthritis, and discovering means of prevention and cure.
      Home and clinic rehabilitation programs for arthritis patients; offered by Arthritis Foundation and by its local chapters.

4. Cancer
   A. American Cancer Society
      777 Third Ave.
      New York, NY 10017

      A voluntary health agency dedicated to the control and eradication of cancer through programs of research, education, and services to cancer patients.

      Special Programs:
      1) Cancer prevention programs offer a variety of programs to help you learn to

detect and prevent cancer. Included are programs to help smokers stop smoking, to help women learn breast self-examination, and to provide screening tests for uterine and colorectal cancer. Contact your local ACS office to learn about the services offered in your community. A pamphlet outlining in detail the steps in breast self-examination (BSE) is available from ACS offices.

   2) Stop smoking clinics

   3) Education and counseling for cancer patients

B. Cancer Care (National Cancer Foundation)
One Park Ave.
New York, NY 10016

Provides information and assistance to cancer patients and their families. Local offices elsewhere in the US.

C. National Cancer Institute
National Institutes of Health
9000 Rockville Pike
Bethesda, MD 20014

5. Depression
  A. National Institute of Mental Health
Public Inquiries Office
5600 Fishers Lane
Rockville, MD 20857

6. Eye Problems
   A. American Association of Opthalmology
      1100 17th St. NW
      Washington, DC 20036

   B. National Society to Prevent Blindness
      79 Madison Ave.
      New York, NY 10016

7. Hypertension and Heart Disease
   A. American Heart Association
      7320 Greenville Ave.
      Dallas, TX 75231

   B. National Heart, Lung, and Blood Institute
      (National Institutes of Health)
      Public Inquiries and Reports Branch
      9000 Rockville Pike
      Bethesda, MD 20014

8. Obesity
   A. National Association to Aid Fat Americans
      P.O. Box 43
      Bellerose, NY 11426

      A nonprofit organization, seeking to raise
      the self-esteem of fat people and to promote
      tolerance toward fat people within society,
      the Association provides counseling to fat
      individuals in such areas as employment, so-
      cial acceptance, fashion, insurance, and

health. It also sponsors research and disseminates public information on obesity.

B. National Council on Obesity
P.O. Box 35306
Los Angeles, CA 90035

A voluntary health agency, devoting its resources to the reduction of premature death and disability caused by obesity and compulsive overeating.

C. Overeaters Anonymous/World Service
Office
2190 190th St.
Torrance, CA 90504

A fellowship of men and women who share the common problem of compulsive overeating. Based on the principles of Alcoholics Anonymous. There are no dues or fees for membership. Local offices nationwide.

D. Weight Watchers International, Inc.
800 Community Dr.
Manhasset, NY 11030

9. Sexuality
A. Educational Foundation for Human
Sexuality
Montclair State College
Upper Montclair, NJ 07043

B. Institute for Family Research and Education
   123 Fourth St. N.W.
   Charlottesville, VA 22901

C. National Institute of Mental Health
   5600 Fishers Lane
   Bethesda, MD 20857

D. Sex Information Education Council of the US (SIECUS)
   80 Fifth Ave.
   New York, NY 10011

APPENDIX ELEVEN
Organizations—Nontraditional Approaches to Health Care

1. Acupuncture
   A. National Acupuncture Association
      P.O. Box 24509
      Los Angeles, CA 90024

2. Biofeedback
   A. The Biofeedback Society of America
      4301 Owens St.
      Denver, CO 80220

3. Chiropractic
   A. American Chiropractic Association
      Executive Offices
      1916 Wilson Blvd.
      Arlington, VA 22201 (Local chapters)

4. Massage
    A. The American Massage & Therapy Association, Inc.
       152 W. Wisconsin Ave.
       Milwaukee, WI 53203

       This is a nonprofit organization with chapters and individual members in the US and Canada. It provides listings of individual massage therapists in local areas.

    B. The Swedish Institute School of Massage
       875 Avenue of the Americas
       New York, NY 10001

       An accredited school for massage in New York City, founded in 1916. The school trains practitioners to practice massage as a healing technique. Courses in human anatomy are one aspect of the training.

5. Osteopathy
    A. The American Osteopathic Association
       212 E. Ohio St.
       Chicago, IL 60611

       This organization prepares a semiannual fact sheet concerning issues relating to osteopathy. This fact sheet is available free of charge.

APPENDIX TWELVE
Retirement—Agencies and Programs

A. American Association for Retired Persons
   (AARP)
   1909 K St. N.W.
   Washington, DC 20049

B. National Council on the Aging, Inc.
   600 Maryland Ave. S.W.
   Washington, DC 20002

   1) National Institute of Work and Retirement

   2) Pre-retirement Planning Project

APPENDIX THIRTEEN
Social Security, Medicare, Medicaid—General Information

1. Social Security
   Social Security is an insurancelike program which provides workers, workers' families, or workers' survivors with monthly income. Eligibility for Social Security is determined by a worker's contribution into the Social Security system, based on his or her past work history. The exact amount of Social Security for which you are eligible depends upon your age or your spouse's age, the amount of years worked, and average earnings over the last five years of your employment. All recipients of Social Security

over 65 are automatically eligible for Medicare (see section on Medicare below).

As you approach retirement age, the Social Security Administration will provide you with a preretirement interview in order to determine your insured status. Contact your local Social Security office at least three months prior to retirement, after the death of a spouse, or if someone in your family becomes disabled. You can receive Social Security as early as age 62; however, if you wait until age 65, the monthly benefits will be greater.

The Social Security system presents some particular problems for older women. For example, because it is based on earnings, and women have traditionally earned less money than men, female retirees thus receive lower benefits than their male counterparts. In addition, a woman accustomed to living on the combined income from her husband's as well as her own Social Security check is faced with a dramatic change in financial status if her husband should die. She would receive only one check: the higher of the two amounts.

A surviving divorced woman, aged 60 and over, can also receive survivor's benefits from the Social Security Administration, but only if she was married to the deceased worker for at least ten years. If a survivor is under age 60 but has in her care a child under age 18, she is eligible for survivor's benefits until the child's 19th birthday.

Listings for local Social Security offices can be found in your telephone directory under "United States Government."

2. Medicare

Medicare is a national health insurance program for people who are age 65 or older or for people who are blind or disabled. It is a two-part program which pays for part of hospital and medical expenses. All people entitled to Social Security are automatically eligible for Medicare.

Part A: provides hospital benefits to help pay for costs of room, board, skilled nursing, operating room charges, laboratory fees, drugs furnished by the hospital, and rehabilitation.

Part B: an optional medical insurance program, available to Social Security recipients to pay for doctor fees as well as for other health care bills. Requires beneficiaries to pay a monthly premium subject to yearly fiscal adjustment. As of January 1984, the monthly payment is $14.60 per month.

If you do not need or want Part B, so specify on the application form. For instance, some people have adequate coverage continued from a previous job or from a spouse's policy, and therefore do not require additional coverage.

To apply for Medicare, visit your local Social Security office at least three months before your 65th birthday; or if a family member or yourself should become disabled. Bring your birth certificate or other proof of age with you for your initial intake interview.

Local Social Security office locations and telephone numbers can be found in your local telephone directory listed under "United States Government."

For further information on Medicare, write to the following organization for the booklet, *Information on Medicare & Health Insurance for Older People:*

American Association of Retired Persons (AARP)
1909 K St. N.W.
Washington, DC 20049

3. Medicaid
Medicaid, a joint Federal/State/Local program designed to provide financial assistance for medical services to low-income Americans, is administered by State governments based on standards and regulations set by the Federal government.

The types of services, as well as eligibility requirements, are determined state by state based on broad Federal guidelines. Services provided through the Medicaid program nationwide include: short- and long-term care; diagnostic services; some preventative and rehabilitative care; costs of medication; medical supplies and equipment; etc. Once again, however, benefits will vary from state to state.

Eligibility is based on an individual's or family's financial need. Although eligibility is not based on age, Medicaid does help older people to supplement their health care costs for ambulatory medical services as well as for residence and skilled nursing services provided in long-term health care facilities. It is especially beneficial to older persons in need of nursing home care who have exhausted their Medicare benefits and/or other financial resources.

Application for Medicaid is made through the State Department of Social Services. Local offices are listed in your telephone directory. If you think that you might be eligible for Medicaid, call your local Social Services office. The application process can be a lengthy one, so give yourself ample time, if possible.

If you have applied to Medicaid, and your application is denied, you are allowed to file for a "Fair Hearing" by an administrative officer at the Department of Social Services.

For further information about Medicaid, contact your local senior citizen center, Office for the Aging, Department of Social Services, or a local political representative.

APPENDIX FOURTEEN
Transportation—General Information

Transportation programs for older people vary from state to state. Information on what programs exist in your area can be obtained through your local Department for the Aging.

Most states have a half-fare program for people over 65. To be eligible you generally must be a permanent resident of the locality in which you reside and be retired or work less than twenty hours per week. In metropolitan areas, half-fare transport on buses or subways may be restricted to non-rush hour travel.

For information on how to apply for reduced-fare transportation, check with your nearest Department for the Aging office.

Many towns and cities in the US provide so-called Ambi-Wagons to transport ambulatory patients, 65 or older, to and from doctors', dentists', or other health professionals' offices at low or no cost. A call to the telephone number of the local service brings a vehicle to your door. The driver or an aide is prepared to help you get safely into and out of the van or wagon. Locally, senior centers can direct you to this service, or call the Department for the Aging.

APPENDIX FIFTEEN
Volunteer Opportunities—Agencies and Programs

A. ACTION
   806 Connecticut Ave. N.W.
   Washington, DC 20525

   Regional offices in large urban centers.

   1) Foster Grandparents Program
      Pays small salary to low-income persons.

2) Peace Corps
   Expenses and readjustment allowances.
   Human services provided in foreign
   countries.
3) R.S.V.P. (Retired Senior Volunteer
   Program)
   For retired and semiretired persons 60
   and over. Provides volunteers for a
   wide variety of community needs.
4) Senior Companions
   Pays small salary to low-income persons. Provides care and companionship
   to frail elderly.
5) VISTA (Volunteers in Service to America)
   Expenses and readjustment allowances.
   Provides service to community organizations and social service agencies in
   the United States, Puerto Rico, the Virgin Islands, and Guam.

B. Administration on Aging
   US Department of Health and Human
      Services
   200 Independence Ave. S.W.
   Washington, DC 20201

   Legal services to the elderly. Training provided; legal background not required.

C. American Association for Retired Persons
   (AARP)

Tax Aide Program
1909 K St. N.W.
Washington, DC 20049

Trains volunteers to provide tax counseling.

D. International Executives Service Corps
622 Third Ave.
New York, NY 10017

Counsels overseas business projects.

E. Literacy Volunteers of America
404 Oak St.
Syracuse, NY 13203

Trained volunteers provide tutoring in basic
reading and English as a second language.

F. SCORE (Senior Corps of Retired
Executives)
US Small Business Administration
822 15th St. N.W.
Washington, DC 20005 (Local offices)

Volunteer retired executives counsel small
businesses.

In addition, local hospitals, libraries, day
care and senior centers, and other institutions welcome and often train volunteers.

APPENDIX SIXTEEN
Widowhood—Agencies and Programs

A. American Association of Retired Persons (AARP)
   Widowed Persons Service
   1909 K St. N.W.
   Washington, DC 20049

   Locally, inquire from funeral directors or religious organizations for widow-to-widow programs in your area.

Albanese, A. "Calcium Nutrition in the Elderly." *Postgraduate Medicine* (March 1978).

Alpaugh, P., and Harvey, M. *Counseling the Older Adult: A Training Manual.* Los Angeles: University of Southern California Press, 1978.

Altman, L. K. "The Doctor's World" (column). *New York Times*, June 24, 1980.

American Heart Association. Committee Report. "Rationale of the Diet-Heart Statement of the American Heart Association." *Circulation* (April 1982).

American Osteopathic Association. *Osteopathic Medicine.* Pamphlet.

Anonymous. *Arthritis: The Basic Facts.* New York: The Arthritis Foundation, 1979.

Anonymous. *The Dementias: Hope through Research.* Bethesda, MD: NIH, March 1981.

Anonymous. *Everything Doesn't Cause Cancer.* Bethesda, MD: NCI, 1980.

Anonymous. "Exercising Tips." *New York Times*, September 9, 1980.

Anonymous. *The Heart and Blood Vessels.* Dallas: The American Heart Association, 1973.

Anonymous. *An Older Person's Guide to Cardiovascular Health.* Dallas: The American Heart Association, 1981.

Anonymous. *Psychosocial Needs of the Aged.* Los Angeles: Ethel Percy Andrus Gerontology Center, University of Southern California Press, 1973.

Anonymous. "Purchase of DMSO Stirs Fears." *New York Times,* September 25, 1982.

Anonymous. "Senility: Myth or Madness." Bethesda, MD: National Institute on Aging, NIH, October 1980.

Anonymous. "Sex Roles, Equality, and Mental Health." *Professional Psychology* (February 1981).

Anonymous. *The Silent Process: Essential Hypertension under Control.* New York: Media Medica, 1969.

Anonymous. *So You Have . . . Osteoarthritis.* Atlanta: The Arthritis Foundation, 1979.

Atchley, R. C. "Selected Social and Psychological Differences between Men and Women in Later Life." *Journal of Gerontology* (March 1976).

Basmajan, J. "Tool behind the Catchword." *Modern Medicine* (October 1, 1976).

Beckman, L. J., and Houser, B. B. "The Consequences of Childlessness on the Social-Psychological Well-Being of Older Women." *Journal of Gerontology* (May 1982).

Bequart, L. H. *Single Women, Alone and Together.* Boston: Beacon Press, 1976.

Berg, S.; Mellstrom, D.; Persson, G.; and Swanborg, A. "Loneliness in the Swedish Aged." *Journal of Gerontology* (May 1981).

Bikson, T. K., and Goodchilds, J. D. *Old and Alone.* Santa Monica, CA: Rand Corporation, 1978.

Binstock, R. H., and Shanas, E. *Handbook of Aging and the Social Sciences.* New York: Van Nostrand Reinhold, 1976.

Birren, J. E., and Schae, K. W., eds. *Handbook of the Psychology of Aging.* New York: Van Nostrand Reinhold, 1977.

Block, M. R.; Davidson, J. L.; and Grambs, J. D. *Women over Forty; Visions and Realities.* New York: Springer, 1981.

Blue Cross Association. "Food and Fitness." *Blueprint for Health.* Chicago, 1973.

————. "Stress—A Report from Blue Cross and Blue Shield of Greater New York." *Blueprint for Health*. Chicago, 1974.

Blythe, R. *The View in Winter: Reflections on Old Age*. New York: Penguin, 1979.

Boguslawski, M. "Therapeutic Touch: A Facilitator of Pain Relief." *Topics in Clinical Nursing* (April 1980).

Borelli, M., and Heidt, P., eds. *Therapeutic Touch: A Book of Readings*. New York: Springer, 1980.

Boston Women's Health Collective. *Our Bodies, Ourselves*. New York: Simon and Schuster, 1979.

Bowles, E. *Self-Help Groups: Perspective and Directions*. New York: Center for Advanced Study in Education of the City University of New York, 1978.

Boyack, V., ed. *Time on Our Hands*. Los Angeles: University of Southern California Press, 1973.

Brallier, L. W. "The Nurse as Holistic Health Practitioner." *Nursing Clinics of North America* (December 1978).

Brocklehurst, J. C. *Textbook of Geriatric Medicine and Gerontology*. London: Churchill and Livingstone, 1978.

————, ed. *Geriatric Care in Advanced Societies*. Lancaster, England: M.T.P., 1975.

Brody, J. E. "For Good Nutrition: Balanced Diet vs. Vitamin Pills." *New York Times*, July 7, 1982.

————. "Personal Health Column." *New York Times*, May 28, 1980 (Walking); July 23, 1980 (Fiber); October 1, 1980 ("Bone Loss Is Not Inevitable with Age"); October 14, 1981; October 21, 1981; January 13, 1982; January 20, 1982 (Vitamin C); April 14, 1982 (Cholesterol); April 21, 1982 (Caffeine).

————. "The Science of Dieting: A Fight against Mind and Metabolism." *New York Times*, February 24, 1981.

Brody, S. J. "Public Policy Issues of Women in Transition." *Gerontologist* (April 1976).

Brollier, L. "The Nurse as Holistic Health Practitioner: Expanding the Role Again." *Nursing Clinics of North America* (December 1978).

Brookbank, J. W. *Improving the Quality of Health Care for the Elderly. Conference Report.* Gainesville: University of Florida, Center for Gerontological Studies, 1977.

Brozan, N. "Coping with Travail of Alzheimer's Disease." *New York Times,* November 29, 1982.

Brugess, A. H., and Lazare, A. *Psychiatric Nursing in the Hospital and the Community.* Englewood Cliffs, NJ: Prentice-Hall, 1976.

Burnside, I. M. *Nursing and the Aged.* New York: Mc-Graw-Hill, 1976.

Burtoff, B. "Families: The Role Grandparents Play." *Washington Post,* March 2, 1982.

Butler, R. N. *Why Survive?: Being Old in America.* New York: Harper and Row, 1975.

Butler, R. N., and Lewis, M. I. *Aging and Mental Health.* 2d ed. Saint Louis: C. V. Mosby, 1977.

———. *Love and Sex after Sixty.* New York: Harper and Row, 1976.

Caplan, G. "Mastery of Stress—Psycho-social Aspects." *American Journal of Psychiatry* (April 1981).

Carnivali, D., and Patrick, M. *Nursing Management for the Elderly.* Philadelphia: J. B. Lippincott, 1979.

Cassem, N. H., and Stewart, P. S. "Management and Care of the Dying." *Journal of Psychiatric Medicine* 6 (1975).

Chapman, D. J. "Osteopathy." *Wholistic Dimensions in Healing: A Resource Guide.* Ed. L. J. Kaslof. New York: Doubleday, 1978.

Charles, R.; Truesdell, M.; and Wood, E. "Alzheimer's Disease: Pathology, Progression and Nursing Process." *Journal of Gerontological Nursing* (February 1982).

Chila, A. "Helping Bodies Help Themselves." *Consultant* (March 1982).

Chinn, A. B., ed. *Working with Older People. Clinical Aspects of Aging.* Vol. 4. Washington, DC: United States Department of Health, Education, and Welfare, 1971.

Chu, L. *Education for Rural Women: A Global Perspective.* Washington, DC: National Institute of Education, 1980.

Clark, D. W., and Williams, T. F. *Teaching of Chronic Illness and Aging.* Washington, DC: United States Department of Health, Education, and Welfare, 1973.

Cohen, S., and Booth, G. "Gastric Acid Secretion and Lower Esophagal Sphincter Pressure in Response to Coffee and Caffeine." *New England Journal of Medicine* 293 (1975).

Colman, V.; Sommers, T.; and Leonard, F. "Till Death Do Us Part: Caregiving Wives of Severely Disabled Husbands." *Older Women's League Gray Paper No. 7.*

Comfort, A. *A Good Age.* New York: Crown, 1979.

Corea, G. *The Hidden Malpractice: How American Medicine Mistreats Women.* New York: Jove Publications, 1979.

Crawford, R. "Healthism and the Medicalization of Everyday Life." *International Journal of Health Services* 10:3 (1980).

Dairy Council of Metropolitan New York. *To Your Health . . . In Your Second Fifty Years.* New York, 1980.

Daly, F. Y. "To Be Black, Poor, Female and Old." *Freedomways* (April 1976).

Datan, N., and Rodeheaver, D. *Dirty Old Women: The Emergence of the Sensuous Grandmother.* San Francisco: American Psychological Association Annual Convention, August 1977.

Davis, L. J., and Brody, E. M. *Rape and Older Women.* United States Department of Health, Education, and Welfare—Alcohol, Drug Abuse and Mental Health

Administration, 1979.

de Beauvoir, S. *The Coming of Age.* New York: Warner Books, 1970.

DeGooyer, J. "Older Working Women Face Age, Sex Discrimination." *Generations, Journal of the Western Gerontological Society* 6:4 (1982).

Dickelman, N. *Primary Health Care of the Well Adult.* New York: McGraw-Hill, 1977.

Dietsche, L., and Pollman, J. "Alzheimer's Disease: Advances in Clinical Nursing." *Journal of Gerontological Nursing* (February 1982).

Dinnar, U.; Beal, M.; Goodridge, J.; Johnston, W.; Karni, Z.; Mitchel, F.; Upledger, J.; and McConnel, D. "Description of Fifty Diagnostic Tests Used with Osteopathic Manipulation." *Journal of the American Osteopathic Association* (January 1982).

Downy, G. *The Massage Book.* New York: Random House, 1972.

Edelson, E. "Hope for Breast Cancer." *New York Daily News,* February 1, 1982.

Ehrenreich, B., and English, D. *Complaints and Disorders: The Sexual Politics of Sickness.* Glass Mountain Pamphlet No. 2. Old Westbury, NY: Feminist Press, 1973.

Erdwins, C. J.; Mellinger, J. C.; and Tyer, Z. E. "A Comparison of Different Aspects of Self-Concept for Young, Middle-Aged, and Older Women." *Journal of Clinical Psychology* 37:3.

Erikson, E. H. *Childhood and Society.* New York: W. W. Norton, 1963.

Federal Council on the Aging. "Commitment to a Better Life." *National Policy Concerns for Older Women.* Washington, DC, 1975.

Fein, J. *Are You a Target? A Guide to Self-Protection, Personal Safety, and Rape Prevention.* Belmont, CA: Wadsworth, 1981.

Fengler, A. P., and Goodrich, N. "Wives of Elderly Disabled Men: The Hidden Patients." *Gerontologist* 19:2 (1979).

Fergusen, D. "Biofeedback and Behavioral Medicine: Prospects for the 1980's." *American Journal of Clinical Biofeedback* (Spring/Summer 1981).

Finch, C. E., and Hayflick, L., eds. *Handbook of the Biology of Aging*. New York: Van Nostrand Rheinhold, 1971.

Fink, J. W. "The Challenge of High Blood Pressure Control." *Nursing Clinics of North America* (June 1981).

Frankel, L. J., and Richard, B. B. *Be Alive as Long as You Live*. New York: Lippincott and Crowell, 1980.

Franta, J. "Massage Techniques: Which One Is Right for You?" *Yoga Journal* (September/October 1982).

Fries, J. F. *Arthritis: A Comprehensive Guide*. Reading, MA: Addison-Wesley, 1982.

Fuller, M. M., and Martin, C. A. *The Older Woman*. Springfield, IL: Charles C. Thomas, 1980.

Gambrell, R. D., and Greenblatt, R. "Hormone Therapy for the Menopause." *Geriatrics* (July 1981).

Gartner, A., and Reissman, F. *Self-Help in the Human Services*. San Francisco: Jossey-Bass, 1977.

George, L. K., and Bearon, L. *Quality of Life in Older Persons*. New York: Human Sciences Press, 1980.

Gifford, A., and Golde, P. "Self-Esteem in an Aging Population." *Journal of Gerontological Social Work* (Fall 1978).

Glaze, B. "One Woman's Story." *Journal of Gerontological Nursing* (February 1982).

Glickman, S., and Lipshutz, J. *Your Health and Aging*. New York: Division of Gerontology, Urban Health Affairs, New York University Medical Center, 1981.

Glosser, R. *Meeting the Needs of Rural Women: An Emerging Area of Concern for the 1980's*. Fourth Annual Meeting of the Association for Humanistic Sociology, Johnstown, PA, October 1979.

Glover, B. H. "Sex Counseling of the Elderly." *Hospital Practice* (June 1977).

Glowack, G. "Post Menopausal GYN Problems." *The Geriatric Patient*. Ed. W. Reichel. New York: H. P. Books, 1978.

Gordon, J. "Holistic Medicine: Toward A New Medical Model." *Journal of Clinical Psychology* (March 1981).

Gordon, M. *Old Enough to Feel Better: A Medical Guide for Seniors*. Radnor, PA: Chilton, 1981.

Grabel, W. "Just by Watching Their Salt, 60% Able to Control High Blood Pressure." *Medical Tribune* (April 9, 1980).

Gray, C. "Osteopathy: Is There a Place in Canadian Medicine?" *Canadian Medical Association Journal* (July 1, 1981).

Green, E. "Biofeedback." *Wholistic Dimensions in Healing*. Ed. L. J. Kaslof. New York: Doubleday, 1978.

Green, E., and Green, A. *Beyond Biofeedback*. San Francisco: Robert Briggs Associates, 1977.

Greenman, P. "Osteopathic Medicine—Origins and Outlook." *Postgraduate Medicine* (November 1980).

Haldeman, S. *Modern Developments in the Principles and Practice of Chiropractic*. East Norwalk, CT: Appleton-Century-Crofts, 1980.

Hall, M. R. P.; MacLennan, W. V.; and Lye, M. D. W. *Medical Care of the Elderly*. New York: Springer, 1978.

Hanson, I. *Outwitting Arthritis*. Berkeley, CA: Creative Arts Books, 1981.

Hartman, J.B. *Breast Exams: What You Should Know*. Bethesda, MD: NCI, 1980.

Hayter, J. "Helping Families of Patients with Alzheimer's Disease." *Journal of Gerontological Nursing* (February 1982).

Henderson, V., and Nite, G. "Massage, Therapeutic Exercise, and Pressure for Circulatory and Sedative Effects and Improvement of Muscle Tone." *Principles and Practices of Nursing.* 2d ed. New York: Macmillan, 1978.

Hessel, D., ed. *Maggie Kuhn on Aging.* Philadelphia: Westminster Press, 1977.

Holden, K.; Johnson, A.; and Somers, G. *Monographs on Aging.* Madison: University of Wisconsin Press, 1979.

Hoonyman, N. R. "Mutual Help Organizations for Rural Older Women." *Educational Gerontology* (October 1980).

Hopkins, H. "Speaking Out on Fortifying Foods." *FDA Consumer* (December 1978/January 1979).

Hume, S. *Basic Course in Gerontology.* Albany: New York State Office for the Aging, 1976.

Hungerford, M. "Massage, Oldest Modality of Physical Therapy." *The Massage Journal.*

Huyck, M. H. *Growing Older.* Englewood Cliffs, NJ: Prentice-Hall, 1974.

Isselbacher, K.; Adams, R.; Braunwald, E.; Petersdorf, O.; and Wilson, J. *Harrison's Principles of Internal Medicine.* 9th ed. New York: McGraw-Hill, 1980.

Jacobs, R. H. *Life after Youth, Female, 40 What Next.* Boston: Beacon Press, 1979.

————. "The Typology of Older American Women." *Social Policy* (November/December 1976).

Jauch, T. "Some Causes of Oppression of Elders." *The Elders Speak.* Seattle: Rational Island Publishers, 1981.

Johnson, G. T., and Goldfinger, S. E. *The Harvard Medical School Health Letter.* Cambridge, MA: Harvard University Press, 1981.

Journal of Gerontological Nursing. Special issue on Alzheimer's disease (February 1982.)

Kavanaugh, J. F. "Culture, Value, Formation, and Advertising." Paper presented at the Inter-American Conference of Religious, November 1980.

Kayne, R., ed. *Drugs and the Elderly*. Rev. ed. Los Angeles: University of Southern California Press, 1980.

Kayser-Jones, J. S. *Old, Alone, and Neglected*. Berkeley: University of California Press, 1981.

Kerschner, P. A., ed. *Advocacy and Age: Issues, Experiences, Strategies*. Los Angeles: University of Southern California Press, 1976.

Kivett, V. R. "Discriminators of Loneliness among the Rural Elderly: Implications for Interventions." *Gerontologist* 19:1 (1979).

Kline, C. "The Socialization Process of Women." *Gerontologist* (December 1975).

Koten, John. "Aged and Alone: Many Elderly Women Fight Ill Health, Fear of Crime, Loneliness." *Wall Street Journal*, October 17, 1978.

Krieger, D. "The Potential Use of Therapeutic Touch in Healing." *Wholistic Dimensions in Healing: A Resource Guide*. Ed. L. Kaslof. Garden City, NY: Doubleday, 1978.

——. *The Therapeutic Touch: How to Use Your Hands to Help or Heal*. Englewood Cliffs, NJ: Prentice-Hall, 1979.

Krieger, D.; Peper, E.; and Ancoli, S. "Therapeutic Touch: Searching for Evidence of Physiological Change." *American Journal of Nursing* (April 1979).

Krupnick, J. L. "Stress Response Syndromes—Recurrent Themes." *Archives of General Psychiatry* (April 1981).

Kurta, S. "UTI in the Elderly: Seeking Solutions for Special Problems." *Geriatrics* (October 1980) .

Kushner, R. *If You've Thought about Breast Cancer. . . .* Kensington, MD: Women's Breast Cancer Advisory Center, Inc., 1980.

Lamy, P. P. "What the Physician Should Keep in Mind When Prescribing Drugs for an Elderly Patient." *Geriatrics* (May 1977).

Lapkoff, S., and Fierst, E. *Working Women, Marriage, and Retirement.* Washington, DC: President's Commission on Pension Policy, 1980.

La Porte, H. "Reversible Causes of Dementia: A Nursing Challenge." *Journal of Gerontological Nursing* (February 1982).

Lappe, M. *Diet for a Small Planet.* New York: Ballantine Books, 1971.

Lenhart, D. G. "The Use of Medications in the Elderly Population." *Nursing Clinics of North America* (March 1976).

Leonard, F. "The Disillusionment of Divorce for Older Women." *Older Women's League Gray Paper No. 6.*

Levy, S. M. "The Adjustment of the Older Woman: Effects of Chronic Ill Health and Attitudes Toward Retirement." *International Journal of Aging and Human Development* 12:2 (1980).

Lieberman, M., Borman, L., and associates. *Self-Help Groups for Coping with Crisis.* San Francisco: Jossey-Bass, 1979.

Long, J. W. *The Essential Guide to Prescription Drugs.* New York: Harper and Row, 1977.

LoPata, H. Z. *Women as Widows: Support Systems.* New York: Elzevier North Holland, 1979.

Louie, E. "Working Out." *New York Times Magazine,* August 30, 1981.

Luckmann, J., and Sorensen, K. *Medical-Surgical Nursing.* Philadelphia: W. B. Saunders, 1974.

Macrae, J. "Therapeutic Touch in Practice." *American Journal of Nursing* (April 1979).

McCuan, E. K., and Durn, T. *The Surviving Majority: Older Women and Their Health.* Washington, D.C.: American Public Health Association, 1981.

Maloney, J. P., and Bertz, C. "Aging and Memory Loss." *Journal of Gerontological Nursing* (July 1982).

Marcinek, M. B. "Hypertension: What It Does to the

Body." *American Journal of Nursing* (May 1980).

Matthews, S. H. *The Social World of Old Women*. Beverly Hills, CA: Sage Publications, 1979.

Mayer, T. R. "UTI in the Elderly: How to Select Treatment." *Geriatrics* (March 1980).

Metropolitan Life Insurance Company. "Exercise." *Stay Well Series*. Health and Safety Division, 1979.

———. "Stress and Your Health." *Stay Well Series*. Health and Safety Division, 1980.

Milo, N. *The Care of Health in Communities, Access for Outcasts*. New York: Macmillan, 1975.

Nahemow, L. *Casebook in Geriatrics*. Washington, D.C.: United States Department of Health and Human Services, Administration on Aging, 1980.

Napoli, M. "Non-Medical Therapies." *Health Facts*. Woodstock, NY: Overlook Press, 1981.

———, ed. "Heart Disease." *Health Facts*. New York: The Center for Medical Consumers and Health Care Information, Inc., November/December, 1979.

Nassau, J. B. *Choosing a Nursing Home*. New York: Funk and Wagnalls, 1975.

National Action Forum for Older Women. *Forum*. Stonybrook, NY: SUNY School of Allied Health Professions, 1978.

National Commission on Observance of International Women's Year. *Older Women: A Workshop Guide*. Washington, D.C.: 1977.

National Institute on Aging Task Force. "Senility Reconsidered: Treatment Possibilities for Mental Impairment in the Elderly." *Journal of the American Medical Association* (July 18, 1980).

National Institutes of Health Consensus Development Conference Summary. *Estrogen Use and Postmenopausal Women*. National Institute on Aging (NIH), September 1979.

National Organization for Women Task Force on Older

Women. *Age Is Becoming.* (An annotated bibliography on women and aging.) Berkeley: Interface Bibliographers, 1976.

National Research Council of the National Academy of Sciences. *Diet, Nutrition and Cancer.* Washington, DC: National Academy Press, 1982.

Natow, A., and Heslin, J.-A. *Geriatric Nutrition.* Boston: CBI Publishing, 1980.

New York State Osteopathic Society. *Fact Sheet.* New York: American Osteopathic Association Editorial Department, May 1982.

Notman, M. T., and Naddson, C. C. *The Woman Patient. Medical and Psychological Interfaces.* Vol. I. New York: Plenum Press, 1978.

O'Brien, J. E., and Steif, G. F. *Evaluative Research on Social Programs for the Elderly.* Washington, DC: United States Department of Health, Education, and Welfare, 1973.

O'Brien, P. *The Woman Alone.* New York: New York Times Book Company, 1973.

O'Hara-Devereaux, M.; Andrews, L.; and Scott, C., eds. *Eldercare: A Practical Guide to Clinical Geriatrics.* New York: Grune and Stratton, 1981.

Padus, E. *The Woman's Encyclopedia of Health and Natural Healing.* Emmaus, PA: Rodale Press, 1981.

Paffenbarger, R., and Hyde, R. "Exercise as a Protection against Heart Attack." *New England Journal of Medicine* (May 1980).

Pegels, C. C. *Health Care and the Elderly.* Rockville, MD: Aspen Publications, 1980.

Peterson, J. A. *On Being Alone.* Washington, DC: NRTA/AARP, 1980.

Poon, L., ed. *Aging in the 1980's: Psychological Issues.* Washington, DC: American Psychological Association, 1980.

Pringle, M. B. *General Populations, the Aged, and Women.*

Information Analysis Report. Washington, DC: United States Department of Health, Education, and Welfare, December 1970.

Racy, J. "Stress and Human Disease." *Arizona Medicine* (May 1980).

Rahe, R. "Recent Life Change Stress and Psychological Depression." *Rhode Island Medical Journal* (April 1980).

Raskin, A., and Jarwick, L. F. *Psychological Symptoms and Cognitive Loss in the Elderly.* New York: John Wiley, 1979.

Rathbone-McCuan, E., and Durn, T. *The Surviving Majority: Older Women and Their Health.* Washington, D.C.: American Public Health Association, 1981.

Reichel, W., ed. *Clinical Aspects of Aging.* (A comprehensive text prepared under the direction of the American Geriatric Society.) Baltimore: Williams and Wilkins, 1978.

————, ed. *The Geriatric Patient.* New York: H. P. Books, 1978.

Remen, N. *The Masculine Principle, the Feminine Principle, and Humanistic Medicine.* San Francisco: Institute for Humanistic Medicine, 1975.

Resnick, J. L. "Women and Aging." *Counseling Psychologist* 8:1 (1979).

Rich, T. A., and Gilmore, A. S. *Basic Concepts of Aging: A Programmed Manual.* Tampa: University of Southern Florida, 1972.

Riesberg, B.; Ferris, S.; and Gershon, S. "An Overview of Pharmacologic Treatment of Cognitive Decline in the Aged." *American Journal of Psychiatry* (May 1981).

Riley, M. W. *Aging from Birth to Death.* Boulder, CO: Westview Press, 1979.

Rogers, M. *Women, Divorce and Money.* New York: McGraw-Hill, 1981.

Rosenblatt, J. "Women and Aging." *Editorial Research*

Reports (September 25, 1981).

Rossman, I. *Clinical Geriatrics.* 2d ed. Philadelphia: J. B . Lippincott, 1979.

Ryan, K. J., and Gibson, D. C. *Menopause and Aging. Conference Report.* United States Department of Health, Education, and Welfare, 1971.

Sandelowski, M. *Women, Health, and Choice.* Englewood Cliffs, NJ: Prentice-Hall, 1981.

Scarf, M. *Unfinished Business. Pressure Points in the Lives of Women.* Garden City, NY: Doubleday, 1980.

Schneck, H. "Research into Body's Chemistry May Be the Key." *New York Times,* February 24, 1981.

————. "Some Senility Can Be Reversed, Study Asserts." *New York Times,* July 16, 1982.

Schwaid, M. "Advice to Arthritics: Keep Moving." *American Journal of Nursing* (October 1978).

Schwartz, A. N., and Peterson, J. A. *Introduction to Gerontology.* New York: Holt, Rinehart and Winston, 1979.

Scott-Maxwell, F. *The Measure of My Days.* New York: Penguin, 1968.

Seaman, B. *Women and the Crisis in Sex Hormones.* New York: Bantam Books, 1977.

Selye, H. *Stress of Life.* New York: McGraw-Hill, 1956.

Serizawa, K. "Massage." *Wholistic Dimensions in Healing: A Resource Guide.* Ed. L. Kaslof. Garden City, NY: Doubleday, 1978.

Shapiro, J. H. *Communities of the Alone: Working with SROs in the City.* New York: Associated Press, 1971.

Shields, L. *Displaced Homemakers: Organization for a New Life.* New York: McGraw-Hill, 1981.

Shontz, F. C. *The Psychological Aspects of Physical Illness and Disability.* New York: Macmillan, 1975.

Simos, B. G. "Adult Children and their Aging Parents." *Social Work* (May 1973).

Silverstone, B., and Hymen, H. K. *You and Your Aging*

Parent. New York: Pantheon Books, 1976.

Skully, T. "Biofeedback and Some of Its Non-Medical Uses." *The Holistic Health Handbook.* Ed. E. Bauman et al. Berkeley, CA: And/Or Press, 1978.

Sohngen, M. "The Writer as an Old Woman." *Gerontologist* (December 1975).

Somers, A. R., and Fabian, D. R. *The Geriatric Imperative: An Introduction to Gerontology and Clinical Geriatrics.* East Norwalk, CT: Appleton-Century-Crofts, 1981.

Sprafka, S.; Ward, R.; and Neff, D. "What Characterizes an Osteopathic Principle?" *Journal of the American Osteopathic Association* (September 1981).

Steinberg, F. U. *Cowdry's The Care of the Geriatric Patient.* Saint Louis: C. V. Mosby, 1976.

Stephens, R. C.; Blau, Z. S.; Oser, G. T.; and Millar, M. D. "Aging, Social Support Systems and Social Philosophy." *Journal of Gerontological Social Work* (Fall 1978).

Steuer, J.; Bank, L.; Olsen, E.; and Jarvik, L. "Depression, Physical Health and Somatic Complaints in the Elderly." *Journal of Gerontology* (September 1980).

Stoudemire, A., and Thompson, T. "Recognizing and Treating Dementia." *Geriatrics* (October 1981).

Swedish Institute. *Fact Sheet on Swedish Massage.* New York, 1982.

Tannier, L. M. *Communication and the Aging Process: Interaction throughout the Life Cycle.* New York: Pergamon Press, 1954.

Tenenbaum, F. *Over 55 Is Not Illegal.* Boston: Houghton Mifflin, 1979.

Thomas, L. E. "Sexuality and Aging: Essential Vitamin or Popcorn?" *Gerontologist* (June 1982).

Thompson, D. S., consulting ed. *Every Woman's Health— The Complete Guide to Body and Mind.* Garden City, NY: Doubleday, 1980.

United States Department of Health and Human Services.

Nutrition and Your Health—Dietary Guidelines for Americans. Washington, DC, 1980.

———. *Use of Health Services by Women 65 Years of Age and over in the United States.* Washington, DC, August 1981.

United States Department of Health and Human Services, Administration on Aging. *Aging.* Washington, DC, September/October 1980.

United States Department of Health, Education, and Welfare. "Recommendations on the Impact of HEW Programs in Society: Older Women." *Women's Action Program Report.* Washington, DC, January 1972.

———. *Social Security and the Changing Roles of Men and Women.* Washington, DC: Social Security Administration, Office of Research and Statistics.

———. *Words on Aging: A Bibliography/More Words on Aging—Supplement.* Washington, DC: United States Government Printing Office, 1970, 1971.

United States Federal Council on the Aging. *National Policy Concerns for Older Women: Commitment to a Better Life.* Washington, DC, 1976.

United States Senate Special Committee on Aging. *Nursing Home Care in the United States—Failure in Public Policy.* Washington, DC: United States Government Printing Office, 1974.

Van Coevering, V. *Developmental Tasks of Widowhood for the Aging Woman.* Washington, DC: American Psychological Association Convention, September 5, 1971.

Venet, L., ed. *Breast Cancer.* New York: Spectrum Publications, 1979.

Vernick, J. J. *Death and Dying: Selected Bibliography.* Washington, DC: United States Government Printing Office.

Vida, G., ed. *Our Right to Love: A Lesbian Resource Book.* Englewood Cliffs, NJ: Prentice-Hall, 1978.

Wade, C. *Arthritis, Nutrition, and Natural Therapy.* New Canaan, CT: Keats Publishing, 1976.

Ward, R. A. "The Never-Married in Later Life." *Journal of Gerontology* (November 1979).

Warner-Reitz, A. *Healthy Lifestyle for Seniors.* New York: Meals for Millions/Freedom from Hunger Foundation, 1981.

Weherle, G. R.; Peterson, R.; and Woorley, D., eds. *New Space for Women.* Boulder, CO: Westview Press, 1980.

Wells, T., ed. *Aging and Health Promotion.* Rockville, MD: Aspen Publications, 1982.

Wheddon, G. D. "Osteoporosis." *New England Journal of Medicine* (August 13, 1981).

White House Conference on Aging. *Final Report.* Mini-Conference on Long-term Care, Reston, VA, December 10–12, 1980. Washington, DC: American Association of Homes for the Aging, 1980.

Williams, R. S.; Logue, E. E.; Lewis, J.; Barton, T.; Stead, N.; Wallace, A. G.; and Pizzo, S. "Physical Conditioning Augments the Fibrinolytic Response to Venous Occlusion in Healthy Adults." *New England Journal of Medicine* (May 1, 1980).

Williams, S. R. *Essentials of Nutrition and Diet Therapy.* Saint Louis: C. V. Mosby, 1980.

Willington, F. L. "Urinary Incontinence: A Practical Approach." *Geriatrics* (June 1980).

Wood, V. *Older Women and Education.* Madison: University of Wisconsin Press, 1980.

Zerinsky, S. *The Swedish Massage Workbook.* New York: The Swedish Institute, 1975.

A note on the text
Large print edition designed by
Lyda E. Kuth
Composed in 16 pt Plantin.
on a Mergenthaler 202
by Compset Inc., Beverly MA.